INCONCEIVABLE

INCONCEIVABLE

*A Medical Mistake, the Baby We
Couldn't Keep, and Our Choice to
Deliver the Ultimate Gift*

CAROLYN AND SEAN SAVAGE

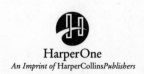

HarperOne
An Imprint of HarperCollinsPublishers

HarperOne

FIRST EDITION

Library of Congress Cataloging-in-Publication Data

Savage, Carolyn and Sean.
    Inconceivable : a medical mistake, the baby we couldn't keep, and our choice to deliver the ultimate gift / Carolyn and Sean Savage. — 1st ed.
        p.   cm.
    ISBN 978–0–06–200463–5
    1. Savage, Carolyn and Sean. 2. Fertilization in vitro, Human—Biography. 3. Surrogate mothers—Biography. I. Savage, Sean. II. Title.
RG135.S28 2010
362.1981'780599—dc22   2010027752

11 12 13 14 15   RRD(H)   10 9 8 7 6 5 4 3 2 1

A Lesson of Love

We have our beliefs.
They may be different from yours.
That's okay, as long as respect endures.
Our story is absent of arrogance, as are our lives.
We realize we may not have it all right.
In fact, that is the only thing we are certain of.
Whether you believe in God, or you don't,
Whether you study the whole Bible, or half the Bible,
Another holy book, or no holy book,
We hope our story will be meaningful to you.
We believe the one thing that we all have in common
is the need to love and to be loved.
Perhaps the purest love on Earth is the love of a child.
Our story is about that kind of love:
Our love for a child,
And the lesson of love he gave in return.

Contents

We have three children. Or do we have four? A strange question, but the kind that parents who have lost a child ask themselves from time to time. That absent child is always with you, a loss you feel some days as yearning and other days in a gasp of pain. My husband Sean and I still grieve the son we lost, despite the unusual way he left us. Or rather, we still grieve him and the circumstances that forced us to give away a baby we thought of as our own. This was a child whom I nurtured and we both protected from the forces conspiring against his survival. Yet I understand that I may never hold him in my arms again and that the next time I see him, he will think of me as a stranger. Perhaps I will never be able to heal the ache that is the place he occupies in my heart. At the same time, I know that if Sean and I had this decision to make again, we'd do exactly the same for Logan.

For us, having children has been the biggest challenge in our sixteen years of marriage: twenty ovarian stimulation cycles, three in vitro fertilizations (IVFs), two frozen embryo transfers, and four miscarriages in the twelve years that we tried everything we could to expand our family. We knew that our struggle was coming to a close on the morning of February 6, 2009, when we entered the fertility clinic for one last try. I was nearly forty years old, and if this attempt at transferring our last embryos did not work, we were done. We would thank God for our three beautiful, healthy children and move forward. Two of my three pregnancies had been difficult, and one nearly lethal, but we were determined to fulfill our pledge to give every embryo a chance at life. Our beloved fertility doctor, who had helped us conceive our third child, Mary Kate, when other doctors had failed, would perform the transfer that morning. Little did we know that, because of a terrible mistake, I would receive another couple's embryos and eventually give birth to a baby we would not be allowed to raise.

All through the Christmas holidays of 2008 and into the New Year, I had been anxiously preparing for this day: taking estrogen pills, injecting lupron and progesterone, and enduring the bloating and grumpiness brought on by those drugs. Although I had started out thinking that I didn't want to go through all of it again, that I was tired of all the anxiety surrounding our infertility treatments and pregnancies, when Sean and I arrived at the clinic we were hoping for a second miracle. I had just slipped on my hospital gown when the fertility doctor entered the examining room. He was brusque and efficient, a man who clearly had many things on his mind as he described the condition of our thawed embryos.

"The five that survived all have developed to between nine and twelve cells. How many will you be transferring today? Remember, I don't do selective reductions."

He meant that if he transferred all five and they survived, he would not eliminate any in utero to give me and the others a better chance. His policy on this was one of the reasons we chose him as our doctor. Besides, I wasn't sure any of these embryos were going to make it. Nine cells after four days in a Petri dish was not robust growth.

"Can you give us a moment?" I asked.

"I'll see you in the operating room. Let me know then."

"Sean, they should be eighty to a hundred cells by now. They are very, very behind. I think we should transfer three. I actually don't think any of them will take."

Sean knew how well I had educated myself about pregnancy, miscarriage, and the science behind IVF these last ten years.

"What happens to the other two embryos?"

"They'll watch them until tomorrow, and if they are still alive, they'll refreeze them. The ones we aren't transferring probably won't survive."

"Okay. Three it is," Sean said.

Before the nurse led me into the operating room, she had me check my wristband to confirm the information there. "Carolyn Savage." "Yes." "Social security number . . ." "Correct." "Birth date . . ." "Wait . . . actually, the day and month of my birthday are correct, but my birth year is wrong. It's 1969, not 1967."

This didn't seem like a serious error, so I didn't think anything of it. The nurse wrote a nine over the seven, fastened the bracelet to my wrist, and escorted us down the hall.

In the operating room, I lay down on the table and placed my feet in the stirrups. Sean came in a few minutes later, gowned in surgical attire.

"How many are we transferring?" the doctor asked me.

"Three," I said.

"We're doing three," he called back into the lab. A few minutes later, the embryologist entered the room holding a catheter.

"You are Carolyn Savage?"

"Yes."

He flipped my wrist over and confirmed my answer with a glance at my hospital wristband, then handed the catheter to my doctor. Sean held my hand tightly.

The nurse squirted ultrasound gel on my stomach and rubbed the wand over my abdomen. Up popped a vivid image of my uterus on the screen.

"There's the catheter entering the uterus through your cervix," the doctor narrated. "Now watch. Do you see that?"

I could see the catheter moving into my uterus, and although I couldn't see the embryos as he released them, I thought of them as light and graceful orbs. I pictured them nesting gently.

"Congratulations. You are now officially pregnant."

I looked at Sean and smiled. Now that our embryos were back where they were supposed to be, they might grow happily.

"That's it, guys. All finished. Good luck. I'll talk to you in ten days, after your pregnancy test," he said as he exited.

I lay still, standard procedure immediately following a transfer of embryos.

"How does it feel to be pregnant with triplets?" Sean said.

I laughed. "Don't look so worried! I know that however this turns out, we'll be able to handle it. Triplets? That would be scary, but we'd survive. Twins? No sweat. A singleton? Perfect! No pregnancy? We'll be okay with that too!"

"Mr. and Mrs. Savage?" A gowned man asked as he entered the room.

"Yes?"

"For your baby album!" he said as he handed me a picture. Sean and I marveled at this snapshot of our three embryos, labeled with my name, Sean's name, and our personal identifying information.

"Their first picture, you know? Congratulations," the man said to us.

Sean and I looked at the picture and beamed at each other.

The First Trimester

CHAPTER 1

The Call to Character

CAROLYN

I ROLLED OVER and glanced at the clock. It was three o'clock in the afternoon, I felt like hell, and I was pretty sure I knew why. I had been pregnant often enough to recognize that I was experiencing those symptoms, but considering my history, I couldn't allow myself to feel certain. Not yet. I knew a virus was going around. The dizziness and nausea from the flu was about the same as what I felt with morning sickness. Soon enough I would get the results of the pregnancy test I'd had that morning. Why hadn't they called me yet? I thought for sure I would know by lunchtime.

That morning I'd rallied long enough to drag myself out of bed, throw on a bra and some sweats, and make a pathetic attempt at doing my hair before hauling myself to a lab for my pregnancy test. It was a chilly February morning in Sylvania, Ohio, and the cold air boosted my spirit as I drove to the appointment at a lab, leaving our sons Drew, fourteen, and Ryan, twelve, to sleep in on their day off from school. Sean had taken our one-year-old, Mary Kate, to his mom's so I could rest. As I entered the laboratory to have my blood drawn, the happy thought that I was about to give her a sibling close to her in age brought a skip to my step at a time when normally I would have been dragging.

Home from the lab, I discovered the remnants of the feast of biscuits and pancakes the boys had made before they went to play with some neighborhood friends. The house was quiet when I drifted back to sleep in our bedroom, enjoying the familiar hormones of pregnancy coursing through my body, with the cell phone and the house phone resting on a nearby pillow.

When I woke at 3:30, there had been no call from my clinic. I felt eerily out of sorts and a little disturbed, as though someone were with me in the room, even though I knew I was alone in the house. Then I had a rush of energy, as if something important had just happened and I needed to attend to it. By the time the clock passed 3:45 and there had been no call, doubt started to creep in. What if I wasn't pregnant? I shivered and pulled the covers tighter around me. I wondered if my shakes were the flu. I rolled onto my left side and felt acid reflux. Why was that there? And I remembered . . . because I was pregnant. Again. I grinned as I nodded off to sleep.

When I woke again as the clock edged toward 4:00, I wondered if I should call the clinic. Surely they hadn't forgotten.

SEAN

IN FEBRUARY 2009, the atmosphere at the financial services company where I work was frenzied. I had been putting in long hours since the markets began collapsing the previous summer, trying to contain the panic virus that was spreading among investors, including some of my clients. Each time my phone rang, I heard my clients' fears; every time I glanced at the computer, the graphs showed global assets in a freefall. On February 16, Carolyn and I were hoping for some good news for a change: the results of her pregnancy test. Carolyn had been ill the night before and early that morning. Perhaps it wasn't the flu, but morning sickness. It was past 3:30, and a call from her was long overdue. My cell phone rang, and I answered it.

"Sean, do you have privacy?" It was our fertility doctor, his voice trembling. *This can't be good*, I thought as I rose to shut my office door.

"I have bad news, but it is not the type of bad news you would expect," he said. "Carolyn is pregnant with another couple's genetic child." My mouth fell open, but words escaped me. *How could that be true? How could that happen?* The hand that held the phone started shaking.

The day before, he said, his clinic's embryologist discovered the error and called him into the clinic, where the embryologist tearfully confessed that he had mistakenly pulled another couple's embryos from cryopreservation. Without knowing, the doctor had transferred them into Carolyn. Our doctor had decided to wait for the outcome of the pregnancy test before letting us know about the mistake. He said he did not have the words to express how sorry he was for the error.

I thought of the day of the transfer, of those embryos floating down to her womb, and then of Carolyn lying sick in bed this morning.

"Does the other family know?" I asked.

"Not yet. I wanted to see what you and Carolyn were going to do. I didn't know whether you would want to continue with this pregnancy. Actually, I thought I would reach Carolyn at this number," he said. "Can you give me her number?"

"No," I said. No way was I giving the doctor that number.

"I think you must consider carefully if you want to continue this pregnancy," the doctor said. "With Carolyn's health at stake and the emotional toll. . . ."

"Call this number in an hour," I said.

After we hung up, I sat at my desk, unable to move. My mind bounced from one urgency to another, like a super ball trying to find a spot to settle. I had to relay this news in person. Carolyn had been my rock, my soul mate, for more than twenty years. We had always done the heavy lifting together; neither one of us shouldered big burdens alone. It was a partnership in every sense of the word. Thinking of how much this would hurt her made me sick to my stomach.

Stand up, grab your keys, and get home, I thought.

I had made the sixteen-minute drive home so often that I could do it in my sleep, which was good, because I wasn't focusing on the road. *This is a life-changer*, I kept thinking, but I couldn't process much beyond that. Mostly I was trying to decide what words to use when I told Carolyn.

As I pulled into the driveway the pounding of my heart shook my bones. I knew Carolyn was in the bedroom resting, and I thanked God that the boys were off at the neighbor's and our youngest was with my mom. I walked upstairs in the silent house, filled with trepidation.

The bedroom curtains were drawn, and the room was nearly dark. Carolyn looked weak and tired in the dim light. I approached her side of the bed, startling her.

"I have some really bad news," I said. She sat straight up in bed. "You are pregnant, but the doctor transferred another couple's embryos into you."

"What?"

"They made a horrendous mistake. Another couple's embryos are inside you. The doctor called to tell me."

"You are joking," she said.

I shook my head no.

She repeated loudly, "You are joking!"

I shook my head no again, and terror flitted over her face.

"You are joking!"

I moved to comfort her, but she flew out of bed. I stood back. She walked toward me with her finger pointed at my chest, as if she was going to make me take back what I just said. Then she stopped. I watched tears building in her eyes, while tears of my own ran slowly down my face. I was her husband, and I was not able to help her. No one could.

CAROLYN

SEAN'S FACE WAS ASHEN and his shoulders slumped, his body drained of his usual confidence. Deep down, I realized he wasn't kidding. As the seconds passed and I understood what he was saying, I lost control.

Sean reached to comfort me, but I didn't want to be touched. I ran toward our bathroom. He followed. I ran from the bathroom to the closet, back to the bathroom, to the bedroom door, and back to the bed, as if I needed to get away, but there was no escape. The problem was *inside* of my body. I realized I was gasping for air. I caught a glimpse of myself in our bedroom mirror. My skin was covered in red blotches, and my eyes were bloodshot and swollen. *Get a grip, Carolyn,* I thought to myself. Then I looked at Sean, who was standing in the corner of our bedroom, tears streaming down his face. I'd only seen him cry twice before: the day his dad died and the day Ryan was born, when I nearly died. Once again, he was crying tears of helplessness. He didn't know what to do for me.

I plopped down on the bed, grabbed my pillow, and hugged it to my chest. Staring at the wall, I tried to catch my breath. I couldn't look at Sean. I couldn't look anywhere.

After a few minutes of silence, Sean moved closer. He hesitated and spoke softly.

"You know, the doctor wants you to terminate."

"What? They want me to do what?"

"He said it would be best for you to terminate."

Our fertility doctor didn't believe in abortion. How could he go against his personal ethics?

I looked up at Sean, and our eyes locked. We both knew what the other was thinking. This was a human life, and we would protect it. It didn't matter that this child was in the wrong womb. That wasn't his or her fault. I put myself in the place of this child's mother. If I were her, I would be terrified that my child's life was going to be taken away because he or she was in the wrong place at the wrong time. What if my unborn child was in the wrong woman? Would that woman be merciful and allow my child to live?

I looked at Sean knowing this was one of those decisions we didn't need to discuss.

"We'd never do that," I said.

Sean nodded his head in agreement. And that was it. We would endure this pregnancy. I looked up at him, but his eyes had drifted to the portrait of our family on the beach that hangs over our bed. I closed my eyes. I wanted to shut it all out. When I opened them again, Sean was sobbing.

CHAPTER 2

In the Name of Family

SEAN

As I LOOKED AT Carolyn, I saw tears running down her face and also felt tears on mine. I could not believe we were in this place. How did our life's journey lead us here? So much of what had driven us since we met was our family. We had sacrificed and spent so much, all for the ideal of having a large family.

The first time I saw Carolyn, at a party that my Miami University of Ohio fraternity hosted in 1989, I couldn't take my eyes off her. She looked just like the woman I had imagined I would marry. She was dressed conservatively, but I noticed a spark, a light she brought to her corner of the room. I asked some friends to arrange an introduction. Up close, I found her in a playful mood.

"Have you ever seen a hair dance?" she asked me.

"No," I said. She plucked a strand of her long blond hair, and I followed her to a beer-drenched table.

"Watch closely as I place this piece of hair into that puddle of beer," she said.

I dropped my head for a better view, and she urged me closer. When I was within a few inches of it, she stretched out her hand and splashed beer all over my hair and face. Bold! I loved that she had the guts to try a trick. *I really like this girl*, I thought.

We decided to go to a party at a fraternity nearby, but that party had ended. I offered to walk her home, and she accepted. We didn't take a straight line back. It was nearly midnight, and the weather was a balmy seventy degrees, unusual for Ohio in October. We strolled up High Street, past the lovely old colonial-style brick buildings that dot the campus, laughing and talking so easily, in our own world. It just felt right. She let me steal a kiss at her door as we said good night.

The following few weeks were a little hit and miss, but by Thanksgiving we were dating exclusively. Two days after Christmas I drove five hours from my parents' home in Toledo to Champaign, Illinois, to see Carolyn and meet her family. All the Higginses were waiting to meet me: Carolyn's dad Byron, her mom Linda, and her brothers, Mike and Andy. Byron was the chief counsel for the University of Illinois and knew how to take someone's measure, particularly where his beloved daughter was concerned.

Linda served an elaborate, multi-course dinner. Afterwards, I was looking forward to excusing myself from the table for a night out with Carolyn. As we stood up to go, Linda urged us to please sit down for dessert, and she set a piece of her famous cherry pie before me. I hate cherry pie. It makes me gag, but the pride with which Linda presented it alerted me to the fact that I'd better eat it if I wanted to make a favorable impression on the Higgins family. I choked down the slice of pie, slipping several bites to their dog Bailey, who waited eagerly underneath the table, and expressed my compliments to the chef. I passed the test. The reward was sharing an "I love you" with Carolyn for the first time as I was leaving.

The summer arrived, and I had a job back home in Toledo pounding nails at a construction site. Carolyn was on my mind most of the time. Nearly every weekend I traveled to see her in Champaign, or vice versa. The commute to visit her was epic. One Saturday in July, I finished work at 3:00 in the afternoon, immediately jumped in my car, still dusty and sweaty, and arrived at her house around 7:30. On Sunday I had to be back in Toledo by noon for a family gathering, so I left Carolyn at 7:00 A.M. I spent ten hours in the car to spend twelve hours with Carolyn.

As our one-year dating anniversary approached, I wanted to give Carolyn something special. On our anniversary—October 29—we drove to Cincinnati, where I bought her a beautiful Irish Claddagh ring. I put it on her finger as a placeholder for the ring I planned to give her in the future. I had no doubt we were moving toward a life together, a life with family at its center. During one happy evening early on, we imagined sitting at opposite ends of our kitchen table with our raucous children in between. We even named them.

In the late spring of 1992, just after I graduated, I got down on one knee in the Formal Gardens at Miami University and proposed. Carolyn said yes, and the wedding plans began within minutes. On May 29, 1993, one hundred days after my father, John F. Savage, passed away, we wed in St. John's Catholic Chapel in Champaign, Illinois. Carolyn joined me in Toledo, where I worked for State Farm Insurance as a corporate employee and Carolyn taught eighth-grade language arts at a Catholic school. Within a few years, I joined Savage & Associates, the financial services firm that my father founded, later run by my uncle Bob Savage. By then, we had two sons and Carolyn was working on her master's in education and would soon be the principal of an elementary school. What could stop us from achieving our dreams?

In a word, infertility.

CAROLYN

THOUGH SEAN FELL FOR me immediately, I took a little while longer. Sure, I let him kiss me when he walked me home, but a few nights later we passed each other on the street and I didn't recognize him. I think there was some beer involved in that episode too. I guess I needed some more time. The first time he came to visit my apartment, my roommate and I were looking out the front window as Sean approached, wearing a shiny blue tracksuit to our first date! She chuckled. "Well," she said, "maybe you can teach him how to dress, 'cause he's even cute wearing that."

Despite our beginning, when I fell for Sean, I fell completely. He is quick and witty, and like me, he never shrinks from a challenge. In each other, we truly had met our match. Besides our ambitions, we shared a faith, the same goals, and, at the center of it all, a desire for a big family. We both thought raising children was the best show on earth. I could spend my entire day snuggling babies, burying my kisses in their necks, and listening to them giggle. We agreed to have at least four children, but I wouldn't have been opposed to five or six, if we could support them. Sean is the eighth child of John and Kate Savage's brood of nine, and his description of growing up in a big family appealed to me.

I met the Savage clan for the first time when Sean and I had been going out for about six months and he took me home for his sister Patti's wedding. As we drove toward the church that afternoon, Sean warned me that I'd be introduced to more than a hundred of his blood relatives at the ceremony. How would I keep all those names straight? Sean didn't make things any easier on me with his stories about his brothers.

"You should be glad this is a wedding and not all of us sitting around the dinner table. My brothers all rate the new girlfriends when someone brings one home."

"Excuse me?"

"Like sometimes one of them will bring home a date for dinner, and we all just shout out numbers while we are eating."

"That's awful!"

"Not really. She never knows what we're doing. We just ask for 'three rolls' or 'seven green beans.' Don't worry. You'd get some high numbers."

Some high numbers? After the ceremony, my mind was tied

up in knots as we pulled into the driveway of the Savage home, which sat amid five acres on a hillside in a suburb of Toledo. The Savages were hosting four hundred guests at a beautiful reception in a hall nearby. Honestly, I hardly noticed the food. Most of my energy went into memorizing the names of all the siblings and their spouses. There was John and Cindy; Kevin and JoAnn; Jeff and his girlfriend Carol; Scott and Julie and their one-year-old, Kristen; Brian and Beth; the bride Patti and her new husband Pat; Kelly; and Sean's younger brother, Aaron.

"Then there are my cousins," Sean said. "My dad has eight siblings." I must have looked dumbfounded. "Don't worry. I don't even know all of their names. My aunts make everyone wear name tags at family gatherings."

This was the large family I wanted for my children. Of course, I had a happy childhood and love my family with all my heart. I have wonderful memories of sailing on Lake Huron in the summers. And our family dinners, every evening at six o'clock sharp, were precious to me. Yet the grand scale of this family captured my imagination. I definitely saw a place for myself among the Savages.

Part of what drew me to them was their faith.

My family was religious but not active in a parish, which was tough for a little girl who liked ceremony and regimen. The Savage family life was intertwined with the life of the church, something I also craved: a community that watched out for each other, linked through the ceremonies of life—the births, the deaths, and the holidays. In Sean's family, all of it was held in place by the power and charisma of Sean's dad.

Revered in his industry, John Savage also was a motivational speaker with engagements all over the world. He easily could have paid for college for all of his children, but he devised his own motivational scheme to build character in them. The kids would pay for half of their college education. On the day they graduated, their father would give them back all the money they had put in.

During our engagement, Sean's dad was diagnosed with an aggressive form of leukemia. He died three months before our wedding, and it seemed as though the whole town went into mourning. John Savage's death was front-page news for three days. There must have been a hundred cars in the procession behind the hearse, which paused briefly in front of John F. Savage Hall, the University of Toledo's beautiful basketball arena that had been named in his honor, a testament to his kind spirit, generosity, and skills as a fund-raiser. The seven Savage sons, including Sean, served as pallbearers.

In big Irish families, life is always moving on, despite the sorrows. The year John Savage died, we were married and a Savage baby boom was under way. We already had nieces Kristen and Meredith, and five more babies were due the year of our wedding. I hoped I'd soon be joining their number, but we weren't certain, as I was already suffering some fertility problems. Doctors had diagnosed my endometriosis when I was a teenager, and I underwent an operation to remove scar tissue caused by that condition while I was in college. Before Sean and I married, my doctor told us that, if we wanted children, we would have to start right away. We took him seriously, and I was proud to be five months pregnant on our first anniversary.

Drew's conception came the old-fashioned way, and his birth went perfectly. We had beaten the predicted—almost promised—problems of infertility. If I had known what was to come, I would have memorized every moment of the day Drew was born. We tried right away for a second child, but it would never again be that easy.

Our infertility treatments began with the most benign techniques: charting basal body temperatures to predict ovulation and trying like hell to conceive at times not at all inspired by romance. I'm pretty sure that our second son was conceived on a Sunday night during an episode of *Murder She Wrote* after an ovulation stimulation shot. Not the most romantic of conceptions, but it worked.

My second pregnancy progressed smoothly until ten weeks

before my due date. Late one night I felt woozy and was experiencing increasing abdominal pain. Sean rushed me to the hospital. My blood pressure had soared to 160/100, and they admitted me, suspecting preeclampsia, a dangerous condition of pregnancy when the mom's blood pressure spikes and the placenta starts to break down. Early the next morning my obstetrician diagnosed HELLP syndrome, a rare and extremely deadly form of preeclampsia. The only way to save my life and our baby's life was an emergency C-section. I delivered our second son at 10:30 that evening. He was underweight and admitted to the neonatal intensive care unit (NICU). I spent the next ten days in the hospital recovering. A month later, Ryan arrived home to meet his big brother—our well-earned happy ending—at a whopping three pounds, fifteen ounces.

After Ryan was born, all the physicians we consulted agreed that HELLP syndrome was unlikely to happen again, and we were clear to try for another child. During the next ten years I underwent an enormous number of treatments. Every now and then we would ask if in vitro fertilization was something we should explore, but our doctors always said that we didn't need that kind of technology. My ovaries responded well, and Sean's sperm were Olympic swimmers.

So what was the problem? Could it be stress? We thought so from time to time. For several years, as we raised our two active sons, I pursued a graduate degree with the goal of advancing from classroom teaching to a position as a principal. Sean was spending long hours building his financial services business. We found ourselves questioning whether we should keep trying for another child.

In 2005 I was working as a principal, and we were seven years into our quest for a third child. With our busy schedules, miscommunication was a constant problem. Something had to give.

One night I had a school board meeting that Sean had known about for weeks. I was just entering the meeting when my cell phone rang. I answered it.

"Hi, Carolyn. It's Geoff Aughenbaugh. I'm at cross-country practice, and it seems Sean left early and forgot something."

Sean coached Drew's cross-country team, and he always left early on Monday evenings to get to Ryan's soccer practice, where he was also the head coach. "Yeah, Geoff, listen. Can you just put whatever he left in your car and bring it to practice with you tomorrow?"

"Uh, not really. He left Drew!" In years past, Drew had accompanied Sean and Ryan to soccer practice, but that year he was old enough to stay home alone. I thought Sean would arrange a ride home for Drew, but with our frantic schedules, both of us had forgotten to make sure that one of us would do that.

I was livid with Sean, and as it turned out, he was just as frustrated with me. That night, before bed, we started blaming each other, and I ended up locking myself in the bathroom in tears.

As I stood there looking at my tired, anxious face in the mirror, I recalled that there'd been a few too many incidents like this recently—too many for my comfort anyway. The week before, when I was driving the boys to school, I was so worried about a morning meeting that I forgot to drop them off. I drove a few miles past their school when Drew said, "Mom, where are you going?" By the time I turned around, delivered them to school, and fought the traffic to my job, I was late. And the week before that another mom had asked me how I balanced the boys' school lunches nutritionally. I confessed that I didn't pack their lunches. She looked at me as if I was the world's worst mother. Her reaction was extreme, and it was none of her business, but she'd made me feel guilty. The truth was that I would have loved to have the time to make their lunches, to know during the day that they were eating something I'd chosen for them, something that would not only sustain them but allow me to touch them in some way at their midday meal. A small thing, but it mattered to me.

When I walked out of the bathroom, Sean was waiting. He said what I'd been thinking for weeks: "You know, you don't have to work. We can manage."

I wanted to slow down. I longed to enjoy our family. But it was hard to fathom walking away from being a principal. I'd worked so hard to get that job.

Once again, Sean said just what I needed to hear: "You could always try quitting, and if you miss it too much, you can go back."

Right then and there, I decided to give it a try. At the end of the school year, I resigned from my position to start my new job as a stay-at-home mom, pledging to myself that I'd pick up my career at some later date. It also wasn't far from my thoughts that without the added stress of two careers, we just might be blessed with another child.

That fall, we headed back to our doctor to try for a third child in earnest. After three more unsuccessful ovulation stimulation cycles, we were verging on hopelessness. By the time we made an appointment to discuss whether there was anything else we could do, we were exhausted. When I thought about being pregnant, I felt like a failure. Prior to the unsuccessful stimulation cycles, I'd had two miscarriages in which the babies died before they even had a heartbeat. We needed something more.

"The techniques we're trying aren't working," I told our fertility doctor. "I make tons of eggs. You said Sean's sperm is fine. Why aren't we pregnant?"

"I don't have an explanation for this. The only remaining option we have left is in vitro fertilization. But clinically, you shouldn't need it."

"Well, obviously we need something more than what we're doing," I said.

"I'm not sure I really understand IVF," Sean said.

"You're familiar with the first part of it, as it starts out the way we've started before. Carolyn would take medications to stimulate her ovaries to produce eggs. When her eggs are mature enough, I will surgically remove them and use your sperm to fertilize them in the lab. Then we wait. We watch the embryos every day to see how well they are growing. Between three and five days later, we transfer one, two, or three of the embryos back into Carolyn's uterus."

"How do we decide how many to transfer?" Sean asked.

"I determine the quality of the embryos, and we talk it over. If the embryos are growing well, I would never transfer more than two. If the embryos are of lesser quality, we might transfer three. What we don't want is you carrying three or four babies."

"After the transfer, we wait two weeks before the pregnancy test," I said.

"That's right. We hope by that time at least one of the embryos has implanted in your uterus and begun to grow."

"Isn't this very expensive? Our insurance doesn't cover the procedure," Sean asked.

"After medications, office visits, and surgical procedures, it will run you around $8,000 per try."

The blood nearly ran out of Sean's face. That was a lot of money, especially considering we had already spent a small fortune over the course of the previous decade on medications for our ovulation stimulation cycles.

The money wasn't the only aspect of IVF that made us think carefully before proceeding. After we left the doctor's office, we had to seriously consider what our Church said about our options. Before we entered the world of infertility, I hadn't thought much about the Catholic Church's stand on this issue; I understood the Church's condemnation of anything that takes procreation out of the intimate relationship between a man and a woman, but I had hoped that IVF was an issue I would never have to grapple with. After all, we were a strong Catholic family, and our choices about how to spend our time and raise our children had always been consistent with our religious beliefs. In addition, I had worked my entire career in Catholic schools, and Sean was raised in a devout Catholic family. Our boys attended a Catholic school, and nearly all of our friends were people we knew from church or school. Considering how we lived our lives, we couldn't lightly dismiss church doctrine on the subject.

Yet after examining the Church's opposition to assisted reproductive technology, we found that stance discriminatory. The Church is definitely pro-family. IVF helps committed couples build the families they so desire. What could be immoral about that? If we followed its underlying logic, the church doctrine was in essence saying that God wanted to deny us a larger family simply because I had a disease (endometriosis). That seemed ridiculous to us. My eggs fertilized fine; they just couldn't navigate their way through the fallopian tubes to implant in my womb. IVF allows embryos to go directly to the uterus. Miraculous technology. God-given technology, we believed.

To us, it seemed like the Church might eventually accept this technology and all the love and joy it brings to couples who want so desperately to bring more Catholic children into the world. Also, it was clear to us that other families in our parish had wrestled with this issue and decided that they did not agree with the Church's opinion about assisted reproductive technology either. Our boys' Catholic grade school was full of fraternal twins and triplets!

After going back and forth on the issue many times, we finally decided to try IVF. We had no intention of ever challenging the Church regarding its stance on it. We just decided to move quietly onward. If God wanted to take it up with us later, we decided, then so be it.

Our doctor was so gracious and understanding as we struggled with this issue, as well as with the questions that remained after we made our decision. Of all the professionals we encountered on our long quest to have more children, our first fertility doctor was among the kindest and most patient, and we are grateful to him for his generosity. He sat for hours with us answering every question we had in painstaking detail. I never left an appointment with him feeling that he thought our questions were ignorant or that he'd become impatient with our inability to decide. Instead, with his gentle, kindly face and honest blue eyes, he gave us the feeling that everything we asked was reasonable and that he would respect our wishes.

Once we decided to consider IVF, we asked for an appointment to discuss how to ensure that the procedure would be conducted in a way that fit our values. "How many embryos could we create in an in vitro cycle?" Sean asked our doctor.

"Successful cycles yield around twelve to fifteen embryos."

We looked at each other. That seemed like a lot!

"Are all of those embryos potential lives?" Sean asked.

"No. Not every embryo develops. Some fail to thrive naturally. We would hope that you would have a nice batch of healthy embryos to choose from at the time of transfer."

"What happens to the embryos that are alive but we don't transfer?"

"They can be cryopreserved, donated, or discarded," the doctor said.

"Well, we certainly can't discard them. And I can't imagine donating them to another family. They are our potential children," Sean said, and I nodded vigorously.

"We'll just transfer every last one of them, until there aren't any more left," I suggested.

So it was settled. We'd go forward with IVF, and if I did become pregnant with that first fresh transfer, we would bank the frozen embryos, hoping they might result in more children at a later date. One way or another, we'd make sure that all our embryos had a chance at life.

When, in August 2006, we found out I was pregnant after our first IVF transfer, we told no one. My new ob-gyn, Dr. Elizabeth Read, suspected I had blood-clotting problems that had probably contributed to our troubles conceiving and the two miscarriages I'd had. We wanted to make sure the pregnancy was viable before we broke the news. She ordered tests to confirm her suspicions. We were so hopeful. With the pregnancy and Dr. Read's new theory, we felt as though at last we'd figured it out.

At Thanksgiving that year we wrapped up an ultrasound picture and gave it to my parents just before dinner. It took them a minute, but when they finally realized what it was, my mom burst into tears of joy. Our boys, then ages twelve and nine, were ecstatic to have another child in the family.

At my twelve-week doctor's appointment to get my blood test results, Dr. Read ordered an ultrasound. I watched the screen eagerly. I saw our baby's arms, legs, and head, and I searched for the familiar flutter of the heartbeat. I saw no movement of any kind. I thought maybe I was looking at a still image, until the technician hastily switched off the monitor and yelled for Dr. Read.

My doctor came to my side when the image went back up. She gripped my left arm, as if trying to stop me from falling off the table. No one spoke. We all just stared at my baby. Finally I said aloud what I needed to say: "My baby is dead."

Bad news has a sound. For me, it pierces the air like a fire alarm, flooding my senses. I called Sean, and he was there within minutes. Dr. Read tracked down the results of my blood tests, and her suspicions were confirmed. I did have two clotting disorders, and she said they probably contributed to my miscarriage. With our next pregnancy, she recommended that I take blood thinners.

Our next pregnancy? I thought that it was absurd to assume I'd ever get pregnant again. We had a new plan of attack, and a few embryos in storage, but first I'd have to achieve a pregnancy, and that was no small task.

After the miscarriage, I entered a world of darkness. I wanted my baby back. I was trying to put Christmas together for my family, but I cried almost every day. With every tear, the wound in my heart

felt bigger. I called my fertility doctor to report the miscarriage, and
we decided to try again in February with the two frozen embryos
left from the previous IVF cycle. When that transfer was unsuccessful, we decided to schedule another IVF cycle in the spring.

The day after our egg retrieval in April, the phone rang earlier
than I had expected. The embryologist's voice had that unmistakable
tone of doom. None of our eggs had fertilized, which almost never
happens. I couldn't believe that the cycle was dead in the water and
our $8,000 check for the procedure hadn't even cleared our bank.

We felt forsaken. We had worked so hard, done everything
right, spent a small fortune, and were left holding empty hearts.
Our doctor couldn't explain the failures. I couldn't imagine walking away after we had invested so much time and money. What if
the next cycle yielded the golden egg? We still had time, didn't we?
It couldn't end with this.

I was wrestling with this when I attended a women's retreat
that was structured to deepen the participants' relationship with
God. Each of us was assigned an area of faith to speak about on
the final day. My topic was discipleship, which meant learning
how to discern and follow God's will. I had no idea how I would
speak about this issue. I am anything but a follower. I am more of
a "do it myself-er come hell or highwater-er." Yet I recognized
that I was at a time in my life when my perspective on things was
changing. I asked Sean to attend my witness so we could discuss
it afterward. He couldn't enter the room with me and the other
women, but he was allowed to listen in from the hallway.

On the first day of the retreat, we were told to meditate on our
lives as we sat in the chapel and to consider handing our troubles
over to God. Let go and let God. I scowled at those words. I thought
"let go and let God" was a load of crap. I was much more in the
camp of "pray to God, but row to shore." Or have a plan and ask
God for help along the way. But something hit me as I sat in the
pew. I suddenly thought discipleship might be a good direction for

me and for our family. Perhaps it was God's will that I not have another child and that I stop draining myself and my family with the costs of a hopeless quest. I made a commitment to myself to be happy and quit chasing my dream of more children. I wrote down my promise to "let go and let God," tucked it in a box, and laid it at the altar as a promise.

Later that afternoon I went to the front of the meeting room to address the other women on the retreat.

"A good disciple listens to the word of God and spreads the good news to all those who listen. But I am not a preacher. A good disciple lives a life that would make Jesus proud, but I am a sinner. A good disciple trusts in the Lord and uses the gift of life to make the world a better place. But I am a dream chaser, running in circles, trying to get what I want from my life. What if my body can't do what I want it to do? Does that make me a failure? Not if I'm a disciple. Not if I listen, surrender, and move on to a better, more peaceful life.

"This morning I folded my dream for a baby in a paper. I folded the dream and gave it to God. If God means for me to have more children, it will happen. If God means for me to have only two children, then that will happen. I am a disciple. I will follow, learn, and move on to a more peaceful life. To do anything else would be shameful. So today, right here in front of all of you, I give up. I'll let go and let God because I am a disciple."

And give up is exactly what I did. For the first time, I believed I had the strength to walk away from my infertility struggle, although doing so made me uneasy. Sometimes the decision to walk away from struggle feels like a release, as if a weight has been lifted off one's shoulders. Giving up on our quest for a larger family felt sad, as if I'd failed. One burden had been lifted, but it had been replaced by another: a heavy feeling of defeat.

SEAN

I WAS NOT ALLOWED in the room where Carolyn was speaking, so I stood in a dark hallway outside listening through a six-inch crack in the door. Carolyn spoke about our experience with infertility, the failures, month after month, year after year, that beat the hell out of us. I teared up as I listened to her close the door on our childbearing years. To have your partner give up on a dream is a failure for both of you. I didn't really want to give up. As I walked down the hallway and out to the car after she was done, hope seemed to be leaving with me.

I was partially to blame for this failure. I'd been the one who'd kept saying our family was fine the way it was. I had not wanted to keep spending hard-earned money when we weren't getting results. I wanted to know when enough was enough. So one would have thought I'd be relieved by Carolyn's words. Instead, I felt sad and guilty.

I remembered our last conversation on the subject a few weeks before as we lay in bed after the boys had gone to sleep. This was our sacred time, when we always talked about what mattered most.

"Drew and Ryan are beautiful and healthy," I said. "Why can't this be our family?"

"Sean, you don't understand. Our family is supposed to be bigger than this. The doctors have never said we can't have more children. Never."

"I am grateful for what we have instead of being sad about what we don't have. We spend more money every month on fertility than we do on our mortgage. We have nothing to show for it but agony and tears. Look at what this is doing to us."

"We are great parents, and great parents should have more children if they want them," Carolyn said.

"I am not opposed to more children. But at what cost?"

Was it frustrating spending so much money and emotional

energy with no results? Hell, yes! Was it hurting our relationship? Yes, it was. For me it was a roller coaster. At times I was really supportive, and at times, needing a break, I would block Carolyn's efforts.

After her witness ceremony, I felt guilty for putting up barriers and partially responsible for this sad defeat. Perhaps there had been one or two golden opportunities that we missed because I was dragging my feet.

Then I found myself wondering if we still had a chance. *If so, I thought, we should give it another shot.* I didn't feel it was my place to urge Carolyn to try again. She'd been through so much already. And of course, it was her body and her health at risk. I had to acknowledge that part of the reason I hesitated to keep trying for another child was this very risk.

My mind drifted back to the night Ryan was born, when I'd made a silent pledge to myself to never put her through a birth like that again. The doctors worked twelve hours to stabilize Carolyn and then rushed her in for an emergency C-section. As I paced back and forth outside the delivery room, I prayed that she and the baby would be okay. Then suddenly the doors swung open, and the emergency neonatal crew wheeled out our little boy in an incubator. I had thirty seconds to introduce myself, and then they whisked him away. Mother and baby survived, but the doctor said that had it been thirty years earlier, I would have walked out of the hospital by myself.

When I finally was allowed to see Carolyn, she was weak and so groggy that she had yet to learn the sex of our baby. I whispered that we had a boy, and she smiled. The sad thing was that neither of us was present for the delivery. I was in a hallway, and she was knocked out. As I walked out of her room, Carolyn's dad pulled me aside and said, "No more babies." Point taken.

Since then, Carolyn and I had convinced ourselves many times that we were done; then hope would return and we would try again.

Now it looked like we were finally done. But I couldn't help thinking that, with a new fertility doctor, we might fulfill our quest.

When Carolyn returned from the retreat, I shared with her how her speech had affected me. We laughed about how amazing it was that I was now the one pushing the idea of trying again. After a long talk, we agreed to give it another shot with a new clinic. It looked like hope really did spring eternal.

Carolyn researched the top doctors in our area, and we made an appointment with one at a practice in Cleveland who had an excellent reputation. As we drove there, we felt optimistic. The receptionist ushered us to a patient room, and when the doctor finally arrived, she seemed rushed and behind schedule. She paged through our file, as if for the first time, while Carolyn sprinted through an abbreviated version of her fertility history. The doctor seemed flabbergasted by our story.

"You've certainly tried a lot of stim cycles without success," she observed. "Why is there such a big gap here in your treatment history?"

This didn't seem relevant. The tone of her voice implied that she didn't understand why we were here. *What in the world is going on?* I thought. I didn't expect that we'd have to explain our longing for another child at a fertility clinic.

"I think you should consider giving up," the doctor said. "Do you really need to have a third child?"

Suddenly she slammed our file shut.

"I'm sorry. I can't help you. Feel blessed with the children you have," she said as she stood up and walked out the door.

The elevator doors hadn't even shut before we looked at each other in disbelief.

"What the hell was that?" I said.

Clearly we'd just had an appointment with the "anti-fertility" doctor. That kind of advice had to hurt the practice's revenue!

Carolyn's dad always says that his surefire way to get his girl to do something is to tell her he doesn't think she can do it. "Carolyn, I bet you can't dock our boat by yourself." So she did it (at the age of eight). "Carolyn, I bet you can't install that snow blade on that tractor." She did (at the age of thirty-nine). "Carolyn, I bet you can't swim five miles in the lake." She did (at the age of ten, behind a rowboat). Proving people wrong has long been a favorite pastime of hers. There are some things she won't do. "Carolyn, I bet you can't rock-climb!" "Uh . . . you're right. No interest." But if her baby were at the top of that rock, she'd scale it in record time.

For Carolyn and me, the Cleveland doctor's rejection was like a rallying cry. There is nothing that can bring two people together like a common enemy. Carolyn began a new search for a doctor who would take our case. I could not wait to send that doctor in Cleveland a Christmas card showing her our three children.

In the first five minutes of the meeting with the next doctor, he said that he knew how he could get us pregnant. He showed us charts illustrating his impressive success rates. As we walked out of his office on our way to the billing manager, I leaned over and said to Carolyn, "We have arrived in the major leagues."

Once the billing manager showed us the fee schedule, I swallowed hard and thought, *He better be really good.*

He was.

Under his care, we had stellar results on the first try. Of the fifteen eggs retrieved, fourteen fertilized, and because of the large size of the batch, the lab froze five the day after fertilization. That left nine to watch. As the embryos grew, three stopped developing, so we were left with six to choose from on the day of our transfer. Our doctor was thrilled with the quality of our embryos and recommended transferring only two since, at that point, the pregnancy success rate had soared to 80 percent. We agreed, and five days after the egg retrieval the doctor transferred two embryos into Carolyn. We assumed that the remaining embryos would be frozen as we had instructed. We were very pleased.

Two weeks later, we found out that Carolyn was pregnant. When she called me at the office with the news, I held in my enthusiasm. A positive pregnancy test was certainly no guarantee of a baby for us. When I arrived home that night, we simply embraced each other and kept the news to ourselves.

I think of the pregnancy that brought us Mary Kate as an eight-month-long prayer. Carolyn and I prayed before every ultrasound and doctor's appointment. Every night I prayed silently before I went to sleep and sometimes spontaneously during the day asking God to keep Carolyn and the baby safe and healthy.

This pregnancy moved through the first trimester nicely, and then came the shocking but exciting news at our second ultrasound that we were pregnant with twins. Carolyn felt in a way that the baby we had lost a year before might be coming back to her. The excitement was short-lived, however, as the day before Carolyn's twelve-week checkup she called me screaming. She was hemorrhaging at home, losing a terrifying amount of blood on the kitchen floor.

I drove home to help, and we soon were in the emergency room undergoing an ultrasound. The news was bad, but not as bad as it could have been. Baby A's placenta had become detached from the wall of Carolyn's uterus, and a blood clot had formed. That baby had no heartbeat, and a pool of blood from the placenta had collected at Carolyn's cervix. But Baby B was resting above Baby A, had a beautiful heartbeat, and was measuring right for gestational age. We focused on the survivor. Weeks of bed rest followed, but we did not care. "Do anything to get to delivery" became our mantra.

Unfortunately, that day came sooner than we wanted—when Carolyn was only thirty-two weeks along. We held hands tightly as she lay in a surgical room for the C-section. Mary Kate was the tiniest little miracle we had ever seen, a major triumph for our family. We had spent ten years trying to get to her, and now she was here and adored. But anxiety was still close at hand: when they weighed her, they found that she was even smaller than Ryan had been at birth. We were so relieved when the neonatal nurses assured us that she was fine and would thrive.

While MK was in the NICU for the month after she was born, Carolyn convinced herself that she was never going to be pregnant again. Her body was clearly telling her that she wasn't cut out for pregnancy. She even gave away all of Ryan's preemie clothes from ten years earlier. I didn't know what to say to her about this, as she knew as well as I did that we had pledged to give all of our embryos a chance at life. I felt our pledge even more strongly after receiving the blessing of Mary Kate. Embryos were still in a tube with our names on it in a cryopreservation tank. Could there be a sister or brother there for MK and the boys?

In October, Carolyn suggested we visit our fertility doctor to inquire about a frozen embryo transfer and thank him for Mary Kate. She called ahead to make sure it would be all right to bring the baby in. She remembered how it had felt to sit in that waiting room pining for a child, and she wanted to be sensitive to those women who would be there. The staff told us to enter through a side door.

Carolyn had dressed MK in her cutest outfit. When the doctor came in, we thanked him for Mary Kate. We eventually got around to the subject of our remaining embryos. Our doctor said that we could proceed with a frozen embryo transfer as soon as we wanted but that, with so few embryos, we'd probably get only one transfer attempt. He suggested that we act quickly, considering that Carolyn was about to turn forty. We took his advice.

So, in December 2008, Carolyn once again started taking pills and sticking herself with blood thinners, all in an attempt to get pregnant. For the first time we were certain that if it didn't work, we were done. But as the transfer grew closer, we became more hopeful. Maybe we would have four children after all.

CHAPTER 3

Shaking Off the Shock

CAROLYN

THE AFTERNOON WE FOUND OUT about the embryo mix-up, I sat on our bed with my face in my hands, trying to contain my grief and my fear. I didn't know what to do next. When I looked up at Sean, I could see the wheels of his mind turning. He's not a man who lingers in his pain; he needs to act, to make a plan.

"You have to call Dr. Read right away," Sean said.

"Why?"

"I think it's best to transfer care of this pregnancy out of the hands of our fertility doctor," he said.

I reached for the phone and dialed Dr. Read. When she recovered from the news, she told me to get blood work done immediately to double-confirm the pregnancy and set a baseline for further tests as the pregnancy progressed. As Sean and I got ready to go to the hospital lab, he called Father Joseph Cardone, a priest at our church who also works as vice president at the hospital, and asked if we could see him. He agreed.

The weather had turned sunny and surprisingly warm we discovered when we exited the house and got into Sean's car.

"I need to call my parents," I said.

"I don't think you should do that yet. We have to be very careful about what we do. We only learned of this a few minutes ago. We need to decide how we are going to handle this."

I knew Sean was right, but I had an overwhelming urge to run to my mom and dad.

"Are you saying we shouldn't tell anyone? How can I do that?" Sean was pulling out of the driveway, focused on the road.

"I'm saying that we should sit with this for a little while. We want to make sure we don't upset anyone needlessly. Let's get your blood test, talk to Father Cardone, and see what he recommends."

The streets were clogged with people on their way home from work. As we stopped at the main intersection downtown, I realized that I dared not look up. We knew so many people in this town. Some of my former students were now driving, or their parents were driving them to errands or school functions. Sean knew many families through his coaching, plus there were the people he knew from work and his clients. If I looked out the car window, I probably would find two or three people waving at me. I didn't know what my face would betray. As long as I kept my head down, none of the people who looked our way would get a hint of the secret we carried with us.

I used Sean's cell phone to ask our neighbor if she could keep Drew and Ryan for dinner, explaining that something unexpected had come up. When she asked what the problem was, I told her Sean had car trouble and I needed to help him out. How many more lies would I have to tell in the next few months to people who cared about us?

Just as I hung up with her, our fertility doctor called.

"Oh, Carolyn, I cannot tell you how sorry I am about this," he said. I could hear the sorrow in his voice, no longer the sound of the confident physician who brought us Mary Kate on our first try. "My wife and I did not sleep last night. We were so frightened by what would happen if your pregnancy test was positive."

I did feel sorry for him, but we were still so overwhelmed. I had no words.

"I love my work and my patients," he continued. "And nothing makes me happier than helping them have babies. But, Carolyn, you must be careful about this pregnancy. You know that a woman at your age, and with your difficult pregnancies, faces considerable risks carrying a baby to term. Do you want to face those risks for a baby that is not yours? You have to think of yourself. And what about your family?"

He and I had discussed all of the risks in detail before my embryo transfer. I looked up at Sean, who was scowling. He gestured for me to get off the phone, but I was immobilized.

"I'm not sure how this happened. I don't know how it could have happened. I only found out yesterday, and I've thought of little else since," he rambled on desperately. "I would not want my wife pregnant with someone else's baby."

Suddenly I was angry. Who would?

"Look," I said, cutting him off. "We will not be terminating this pregnancy. We're on our way right now to meet with our priest to discuss this."

"Oh, of course. I understand," he said. "Talking to your priest is a good thing to do right now. But make sure you weigh carefully the consequences this pregnancy would have for you, both physically and emotionally. If you continue your pregnancy, you will be risking your life for someone else's child. You have to understand, if you go through with this, you cannot keep this baby."

"I've got to get off the phone now," I said. We'd just pulled into the hospital parking lot.

I struggled to get my bearings as we entered Mercy St. Vincent Medical Center, the hospital where so many significant moments of our lives had taken place. Drew and Mary Kate had been born in this hospital. I remembered being there a few months before Sean and I married when Sean's father was dying. All of us—Sean and I and his eight brothers and sisters, with their spouses—haunted the halls for days, sleeping in the waiting areas. We wanted to be together when John Savage passed away. In this family, birth and death were such natural events, swaddled in love and tradition. Where would I place this pregnancy on that continuum? It was a celebration of life and loss, all wrapped in a baby blanket.

Father Cardone met us at the door of the executive offices of the hospital. I was disoriented by seeing him in a suit, a stark contrast to his Sunday vestments. His voice was also softer, more consoling than the booming tone I was used to hearing at church. Sean had described our situation when he arranged to see Father Cardone. As we took our places at the round table in his office, he placed a box of tissues at its center.

I knew he was looking at me, but I didn't want to look anywhere. I stared straight ahead, not knowing what I was supposed to say. My mind was elsewhere, thinking over all I knew about IVF to see if I could remember something like this happening to another woman. In one IVF mix-up in New York, a white woman gave birth to a black baby, but that was a fresh IVF, not a frozen embryo transfer. How could a doctor screw up a frozen embryo transfer? Did they pull the wrong embryos out of the freezer? Did they mix my embryos with someone else's? Oh God, where were my embryos?

Now think. This is a baby. A human being. Some other couple's precious child is inside of you. What if your baby was in someone else?

"I cannot imagine what you are going through right now," Father Cardone said.

I couldn't say anything, so Sean started.

"We have eight months to go, and I'm having a hard time anticipating what those months will bring. What about the other family? And the delivery? And the possible media onslaught?"

"Sean, don't think too far in advance right now or it will be overwhelming," Father Cardone said. "I encourage you not to get

so far ahead of where you are that you are dealing in the hypotheti-
cal, things that may never happen."

He was right. Based on our history, why should we think about
the delivery? The bigger question was what we needed to do tomorrow. Yet my mind could not stop, and I know I wasn't fully taking
in what Sean and Father Cardone were talking about. I heard Sean
ask him for the Church's official position on IVF.

"The Church's stand on IVF is quite clear," Father Cardone said.
"The Church does not approve of procreation taking place outside
of the intimate relationship between a man and a woman. It also
rejects the notion of 'spare' embryos."

"We know that, Father Cardone," Sean said. "That's why we
wanted to give every embryo we created a chance at life. Our belief
in the sanctity of life is what got us into this situation."

I listened as they discussed church doctrine but had a hard time
focusing because the world seemed upside down. Did it matter how
we got to where we were? I didn't think so. I was lost in conjectures
about what the future would hold for us. I pictured ultrasounds
where we would be forced to admire the progress of a baby we were
going to give to someone else. I envisioned a doctor cutting the
baby out and handing him or her to someone else to love, leaving us
with nothing but wreckage.

Okay, stop thinking. Just breathe. Slowly . . . inhale, exhale; inhale,
exhale.

I looked up at the clock. "I have to get my blood drawn," I interrupted.

Sean and Father Cardone looked up from their discussion. Father
Cardone offered to escort us to the lab.

"Science is not the enemy," Father Cardone said as he left us at
the lab. I wasn't sure what he meant by that as I sat in the little lab
chair, laying out my arm for my second blood draw of the day. The
technician strapped a tight elastic band around my upper arm, and

I could see her prepare the needle, but it felt as if I were watching myself in a movie.

The needle slid swiftly into my vein, and the bright red blood filled the syringe chamber. This blood, my blood, would nourish the life inside me. I would do everything I could to make sure that this life grew strong and healthy. And then I would give this life away. How could science have done this to me? No, Father Cardone was right! Science hadn't done this to me. Another human had made this mistake.

One thing I was certain of was that God had not done this to me. I believed in a loving God. I also believed that God gives us free will. The person responsible for doing this exercised his or her free will by choosing not to protect me. Out of carelessness, this person disregarded my safety. No, God did not do this to me. God loved me. God loved my family. That was one thing that I knew.

SEAN

WHEN WE ARRIVED HOME, we had to pretend that everything was fine. Carolyn had asked our sister-in-law JoAnn to get MK from my mom and bring her home where she could watch all the children for the evening. She was the only one who knew we were getting the pregnancy test results that day. We gave her the thumbs-up, and she smiled and mouthed, *Congratulations*. We had to act as though we were controlling our excitement when we were, in fact, suppressing our anger.

When the boys were settled and Mary Kate was in bed, I laced up my running shoes, put on my hat and gloves, and went on my regular evening run. When I run, I am away from the pressures of the day. Without distractions, thoughts rise up, come through me, in a form of running meditation.

I started down the street that leads out of our little subdivision and turned right at the dilapidated barn just across the road, a remnant of the area's farming days. When we bought our house, Carolyn and I agreed that this was the one we would grow old in. Carolyn had had to work hard at persuading me that we needed to move to a larger place. Then we saw this house on nearly three acres of land, which was about as close as we could get to my childhood home. As I ran farther, I thought of my dad, who died when I was twenty-two, and wondered what he might think about our problem. If I could call him right now, what would be my first question? I knew he would give us unconditional love and support no matter what we did. I bet he'd tell me that the decisions were mine to make, not his. He was such a powerful influence on the way I analyze situations, I knew that I'd handle this in a way that would make him proud.

As I turned onto the road that leads to the trail I run most evenings, it was as if the problem was laid out before me on the flat landscape of northwestern Ohio. Father Cardone was right about needing to stay focused on today and not spinning complications out far into the future. We had enough to do getting through the next day. We definitely needed to keep the news private, as we had done with the prior two pregnancies. The prudent thing seemed to be to suffer in silence until we knew the pregnancy was going the distance.

My pace picked up as I turned onto the road that led into the park, originally landscaped as a golf course. The terrain is dotted with small hills and shallow ponds. I chose the short route, only twenty minutes, because I knew Carolyn needed me back home.

Carolyn.

She was going to suffer so much through the next eight months and for a long time after that. The physical part was daunting, but we had great medical care. That part I knew she would find a way to endure. But the emotional part was uncharted territory. We'd been through many pregnancies and terrifying ups and downs with fertility. And even with all that, I knew I'd never really understand the bond she would develop with the baby. Could I help her through it? I'd do what I could, but that probably wouldn't be enough. We would need to develop a support system so that she would be free to go through whatever feelings she had. Getting help would be the best way to protect her.

The day's events raced through my mind. We needed a lawyer, and we might even need more than one. What power did the genetic family have over Carolyn, me, and the baby? We needed an attorney to give us clarity on the family law involved. We needed an intermediary who could protect our identity, at least at first, in our contact with the other family. They might want to meet us right away, but why would we need to meet with them until we knew the pregnancy was going to result in a delivery?

And when the secret got out, when Carolyn started to show, we'd have to explain somehow why she was pregnant but we would not be able to keep the baby. We'd have to tell those around us about the mistake with the IVF. That would be excruciating. The only plausible explanation was the truth. But how were we going to tell everyone? And when? If the media got on to this story, they could get things wrong, and that scared the hell out of me.

As I ran harder, sweat dripped down my face. My breaths became stronger and deeper as I got into the rhythm of my run. The day would come when we would have to share our secret, but that was way down the road. *Try to stay in the present*, I told myself, just like Father Cardone said.

The boys. I didn't want the boys to suffer because of this. They were developing into such good young men, excellent students and very good athletes. I still coached basketball and cross-country at the boys' school, and I didn't want to give that up. I couldn't let those kids on the teams down any more than I could abandon my own boys. Yet if today was any indication, this crisis would probably add substantial hours to my workweek. Well, I'd just have to suck it up and work harder. The tough part would be the duration of the pregnancy: the next eight months. We'd get through it. We'd have to.

As I exited the park and turned home, I slowed down in order to gather my thoughts. I would tackle the family law issues in the morning by talking to my boyhood friend Marty Holmes Jr., who is an attorney. If we needed a specialist, Marty would know who to recommend.

I took my last fifty strides up the drive to our house, overcome with the enormity of all the things we needed to try to control. I stood outside in the cold for a few minutes looking out at the snow-covered landscape that stretched flat and straight as far as the eye could see. The night was cloudless, and above me I saw a sky thick with stars. Normally this sight would bring me serenity. That night, I looked up at our bedroom window and saw the light on. Carolyn was still awake, and I knew she was suffering. Trauma had forced its way into our home, and I had no idea how or when it would leave.

The simple act of opening the front door without using a key made me feel as if I was leaving my family unprotected. Out where we lived, so removed from any dangers, we rarely locked any of our doors. From that night forward, I pledged to lock the doors and double-check them before I went to sleep.

CHAPTER 4

Our Cup Runneth Over

SEAN

As I came into the bedroom, I found Carolyn on the phone with the fertility doctor. Why was she so polite with him? I think my flustered look helped motivate her to end the call. As I was trying to get to sleep, the doctor called on my cell phone again. He was making an impossible day worse. I reached to answer it so I could tell him off, but I decided to let it go to voice mail.

The next day Carolyn remained sick. It hadn't been morning sickness after all, at least not yet. Mary Kate was a little grumpy too, unusual for her. I hoped she wasn't coming down with the same flu that Carolyn had.

That day I consulted with Marty and his associate Mary Smith, a family law attorney, about writing a letter that would formally sever our relationship with the fertility doctor. Early the next day I made the trip to the fertility doctor's office. My nature is to avoid confrontation, but I wanted to be straightforward and end the relationship in person.

I'd saved the doctor's voice-mail message from Monday night, and I listened to it before I went to his office. The message was frantic, and I felt bad that he and his family were suffering so much.

Listening to it again reminded me that we were dealing with human beings and we needed to care for everyone, regardless of what they had done to us. This was a good thought to hold before I sat down with him. I needed to manage my anger and exercise self-control in this meeting. I hadn't warned him that I was coming, but I figured, after all those phone calls, he'd see me right away. Within seconds, he appeared and ushered me into his private office.

The doctor looked like I felt: neither of us had gotten any sleep. His talk was all over the place—apologizing, offering to give us a lifetime of free fertility treatments, and declaring that this mistake was in no way his fault. At one point he even suggested "reverse surrogacy": transferring our embryos into the other woman's body and keeping the baby she delivered. The idea sounded like it belonged in the circus.

I handed him this letter.

Dear Doctor,

You have informed us that three of another couple's embryos were transferred into Carolyn on February 6 and that Carolyn is now with child. We have received independent verification of the pregnancy. The purpose of this letter is to outline a few items. We have chosen not to terminate the pregnancy. We are requesting that you notify the genetic parents immediately. In the notification process we need to have our privacy protected. Please do not provide the genetic parents any information regarding us at this time, only the fact that we have decided to continue the pregnancy until delivery. We ask that the genetic parents contact our representatives, Marty Holmes and Mary Smith, as soon as they want to establish communication with us. We believe this is the most appropriate manner to open a dialogue between us and the other family. Privacy through this process is very important to us. Doctor, although a very difficult conclusion was reached, we believe that it is not a good idea for us and you to communicate directly regarding this matter and we appreciate you accepting this in the spirit it is being made.

Sean and Carolyn Savage

I went through the letter with the doctor line by line to make sure that he understood our intent. He needed to look me in the eye so that he could get a glimpse of what he had thrust upon our family. In the sincerity of his continuing apology, he gave me a few limited details about the other family, including the fact that the woman had a last name similar to ours. His partner, another physician in the practice, had given the other family the news Tuesday afternoon. I was relieved that they knew, but did they want the child Carolyn was carrying? He answered that question indirectly by telling me that the other family had been scheduled to meet with their doctor in a few weeks to discuss doing a frozen embryo transfer.

I stood up to leave, but he had one more thing he wanted to say. "Sean, I owe everything to you and Carolyn." I looked him in the eye and could see he was in a bad place. I was not even close to being ready to accept his apology. I was simply angry.

As I walked to the car, the sound of ice crunching with each step and the cold, dreary day seeping into my bones, I reviewed the conversation. I could not believe that he had looked me in the eye and said that he was not at fault. How could he have said he owed everything to us and yet contend that he did nothing wrong? His heart was telling me that he was ultimately responsible, but his brain was making the counterargument that others under him were really the ones who screwed up.

No, doctor, I thought, *you are responsible for the mistake. You set the tone on how strictly procedures are followed.* Just as we had thanked him for everything he did for Mary Kate's birth, we had to hold him accountable for everything he did not do to prevent this tragic error.

I got into my car and called Carolyn. As the conversation began, I pulled onto the highway and started the drive to my office. I had worked so very little this week, and it was already Wednesday. It was only the third day of this crisis, and I was already falling behind.

CAROLYN

MY NEW RULE WAS that whenever Mary Kate took a nap, I'd try to take one too. I needed rest. I knew that. But every time I put my head on the pillow, my mind would give me no peace. Physically the baby was no bigger than a speck of sand, but it was everywhere I looked.

I thought about being pregnant. I knew I would feel horrid for the next several months. And if I was fortunate enough to carry the baby successfully, I would probably spend weeks on bed rest with my health endangered and our family life disrupted. I could picture the birth, but my imagination stopped when I tried to picture handing this baby to another woman.

Those first moments when you hold your new baby in your arms are some of life's sweetest. That beautiful fresh life filled with possibilities, and you are the lucky one who gets to be the custodian. And for couples who have suffered through infertility, cradling that baby has a feeling of a victory too. You beat the odds. You got around the diagnosis.

Then I tried to picture the next part: my arms outstretched with the baby offered up in my cupped hands. The hands were in empty space, nothing but blue sky behind them, while other hands came to grab the baby, and then my baby was gone, gone forever. I could get as far as the arms offering the baby up, but then my mind would clamp down in disbelief. I could not imagine giving this baby to someone else.

I drew my green afghan—my "blankie"—around myself for

comfort. Yes, I am a grown woman who has a blankie. This one is the third I've had in my life, purchased after I lost the last one on vacation in 2008. I have a favorite pillow too, and I only sleep with that pillow. I also have to turn on a white noise machine in order to sleep. I guess I am kind of a high-maintenance sleeper. Everything has to be just right, and at a time when nothing seemed right, I wasn't embarrassed to cling to these little pieces of comfort.

Despite my angst, I tried to be the best mother I could to Mary Kate, who seemed to be coming down with something. She was not her usual cheerful self that morning. Maybe she wasn't sick. She might have been responding to the fact that her mom was so distracted. I spent considerable time thinking about the mother of the baby I was carrying and how she would be worried. I figured the only way to keep her feeling safe was to communicate with her, but our lawyers advised us to be cautious. Sean's Tuesday conversation with Mary Smith, our new lawyer, was fresh in my mind.

All communications would be handled by our lawyers. Beyond our commitment not to fight for custody, the other family would get nothing but medical information, at least until we were certain that the pregnancy was viable. I wasn't sure I was comfortable with this approach, but how could we know? We had no idea who the other family was. They could be people who would want to capitalize on this mistake and sell the story. They might be dishonest or insensitive, thinking it was their right to force us to terminate the pregnancy. What I understood from the lawyers was that, at this point, the other family and our family were, in some sense, adversaries.

I wanted to think that the other parents were good, decent people, but that hope might be setting us up for disappointment. Maybe they were generous—so generous that they would rescue me and my family from this nightmare by allowing us to keep the baby and raise him or her as our own child. I could love another couple's child. I knew that. It was something I had experienced as a teacher and a principal. After the baby was born from me, wouldn't the baby always be in some sense mine?

As I burrowed under my blanket, I tried to picture the other mother. I pictured her as a tall woman, older and more sophisticated than me, with short brown hair, wearing a business suit. This woman was a powerful lawyer or a formidable businesswoman, I imagined, someone who had had significant successes in her professional life but had never been able to have a baby. I could give a gift like that to a childless woman. There was so much that I wanted to say to her, whoever she was and whatever she looked like. All the while, I felt badly for her. She probably had the same fears. She would worry about her baby's well-being since she had no control over the situation. As strongly as I felt the yearning to keep the baby, I wanted to reassure the other mother that I would treat her baby as if he or she were my own precious child. Every piece of this that was under my control, and each decision I made, would be with the health of the baby in mind.

All of my thoughts about the other couple helped me understand how much this pregnancy had changed my feelings about having another baby. Only a few days earlier, I had been okay with not having any more children, but now I wanted a baby more than ever. Even though I now had to use bifocals to read the ingredients on the baby food jar, and I was bathing Mary Kate in the kitchen sink to protect my arthritic knees, I'd bathe both of them between the coffeemaker and the toaster until they were toddlers, if that was what was necessary. We could still have another child.

Could I still get pregnant? We had embryos that were left untouched in a freezer in the clinic. If I brought the baby inside me now to term, I'd have to wait at least a year before trying to get pregnant again. Then I'd be forty-one years old. Considering my health history and the number of C-sections I'd had, we would have a hard time finding a doctor who'd condone a pregnancy for me at that age. Besides, I didn't just want a baby. I wanted *this* baby. I already loved him.

Sean called from the road. He'd just fired our fertility doctor, and he said the other family now knew of the error. I held my breath.

"Well, what did he say about them?"

Please, God, please, God, let this be good news.

"He indicated they were eager parents."

"Then they want this baby?" I choked on my words.

"Carolyn, I'm coming home."

When Sean came through the door, I was out of bed and standing in the kitchen with my head in my hands. The concern on his face was tender, but I did not want his comfort. He didn't deserve my rage, and he couldn't help me in my sorrow. Mary Kate deserved a buddy, just like Drew and Ryan had in each other, and I wouldn't be able to give her that, not with the baby that was inside me or any other to come. There would be no more to come. Sean tried to hug me, but I pulled away suddenly.

"This is my last pregnancy. After my third C-section with this baby and my history, the doctors are going to say, this is it."

"We will need to speak to the doctors about this."

"The other family is going to get a baby out of this, and we may never get a chance again."

I could see from the look on Sean's face that he had not yet connected the dots between the mix-up and the end of our chance for another child of our own. He was the consummate planner, someone who could project possible outcomes six, nine, twelve months ahead. Yet each day this pregnancy revealed a new problem. How many dimensions did this crisis have? His arms were still open, still holding the space where he had tried to hug me. I saw his eyes drifting over to his BlackBerry, which was flashing with calls from his office.

"You should go back to the office, Sean. There is nothing you can do for me here," I said.

"I don't want to leave you," Sean replied.

"There is nothing you can do to help me!" I said. "Just go."

God love Sean. I know I do. His reaction to me rejecting him and sending him off to work was to find us a therapist. He was right that we were going to have a difficult time dealing with the emotions as they arose. There was no map for this experience, not as there was for a family crisis like a death or an illness. He remembered a therapist named Kevin Anderson whose articles he'd seen in *The Catholic Chronicle* and whose spiritual take on marital challenges he had liked. I'd heard Kevin Anderson speak before. I remembered him as a peaceful, soft-spoken man with a Zen-like quality. He seemed like a perfect fit, as I needed some Zen in my life right about then.

MK had thrown up Wednesday night, but by Friday morning she seemed on the mend. Our appointment with Kevin Anderson was at noon, and I had no choice but to bring her along. I packed her diaper bag, strapped her in her car seat, and made the twenty-minute drive to the church where Kevin had his office.

I toted MK in her car seat into the lobby near his office door. When I lifted her out of her carrier, I noticed she was wet. On closer inspection, I realized the source of her wetness: a total diaper blowout. My precious baby girl was completely covered. Luckily, I had a spare outfit in her diaper bag. I went around a corner, laid her on her changing pad, and began to undress her. As I got her clothes off, the extent of the mess became abhorrently apparent. I started to sweat—five minutes to the appointment—as I realized that I didn't have enough wipes to thoroughly clean her. Just then, Sean came through the door and around the corner.

"Holy s—!"

"Literally!"

I sent him to find some paper towels as I continued to wipe MK down, hoping and praying that Dr. Anderson would be running late. No such luck. I heard his office door open. I'm sure the stench hit him before he even realized we were hiding behind a corner changing the most heinous diaper in the history of mankind. I heard his footsteps approaching, and I wanted to disappear. He rounded the corner as I looked up. "Sean, Carolyn?"

"Hi, Dr. Anderson. Nice to meet you!" was all I could say as I tried to remove MK's blowout from her hair. "I'm so sorry. We seem to have had a diaper emergency." I could feel my cheeks burning.

"Oh, man. Been there, done that. I have five kids. No worries." He smiled, got me a garbage bag, and showed me where the bathroom was.

Kevin was a tall man with broad shoulders, and his size could have been somewhat intimidating if it hadn't been for the sweetness of his demeanor. He had a full head of brown hair that blended seamlessly with his full beard and mustache. A serene and open spirituality was reflected in his bright blue eyes, which seemed to shine with a deep inner compassion for all living things. I could sense this even if I couldn't focus on the specifics of the conversation he was having with Sean. I confess I don't remember much of that appointment.

While Sean brought Kevin up to speed, I became transfixed by a poster he had on the wall facing me in the office. It was an M. C. Escher drawing of fish and birds, with the dark shapes of the fish at the bottom level gradually becoming lighter and thinner as the same silhouette transformed into the outline of birds in flight at the top layers. That was us right now. Sean and I were the fish in the dark at the bottom. This man was as gentle as I remembered him being when I heard him talk, and his voice was so soothing. I hoped he would be able to help us shed our scales and fly away from this darkness.

We left feeling relieved. We had someone to help us. Sometimes I look back on that moment when he rounded the corner and laid eyes on us for the first time, while I was up to my elbows in . . . well . . . shit, and think that it was fitting. We would have a lot more of that to dig out of by the time this mess was over.

By Friday night Mary Kate was so dehydrated that the doctors admitted her to the hospital. (Our cup runneth over.) In the hospital, she lay in a crib as Sean and I looked in. For a period of time our focus was solely on her, and that, oddly enough, gave us a slight reprieve from our grief.

Late that night, after Mary Kate went to sleep, Sean and I sat back in the hospital chairs and looked at each other. How could one week have been filled with so much? We held hands. Then we agreed that Sean would go home to tend to the boys while I stayed at the hospital. As Sean hugged me good-bye before starting home, he asked the one simple question both of us were thinking: "What is next?"

CHAPTER 5

Heartbeat

CAROLYN

MARY KATE HAD BEEN just under three pounds when she was born, and she has always been tiny for her age. She's a good sleeper, though, and slept through the night from the time she was only a few months old. Most moms would have been thrilled by that and would have left her undisturbed. Yet I always gave her a bottle before I went to bed because I believed she needed the extra calories. This was even more important after she lost so much weight during her illness.

As I sat in the rocking chair with her in my arms that first Saturday night after we found out I was pregnant, I held her tightly. MK, our miracle baby, getting stronger and bigger every day. I thought about how much I loved her.

Those snuggles and cuddles were the moments that I cherished, the reward for pregnancy and childbirth. I knew I would never get a moment like this with the baby I was carrying. It was then that I realized tears were streaming steadily down my face, darkening the front of my robe. In the days since the news, I'd had plenty of practice crying quietly in my bed or with my eyes shielded by sunglasses as I drove about town on errands. I didn't want to disturb the world with my tears or to invite any questions. I couldn't ask anyone but Sean for comfort, and he too was overwhelmed. Plus, he'd fallen ill with the same virus MK and I had. All of us were weak and tired, but only two of us knew I held the source of our stress.

We'd known about this mess for only a week, and I was already getting sick of lawyers. I respected them, and I understood that they were necessary and that we were getting prudent advice, but the way this was all shaved and sorted seemed wrong. The language they used to discuss what we were doing was so cold. Mary told us that we had no legal claim to the child that was growing inside me. But my heart had a claim. This baby could not survive without me, but judges had ruled repeatedly that my contribution to this life was irrelevant. How could that be? There would be no baby without me. *I'm not just an oven. I am not nothing to this child. Right?*

The next day, when the boys were at school and MK was playing quietly at my feet, I began researching the question online, trying to find just one legal scholar who backed up what my heart felt. I pored over laws and rulings. It seemed that, in most states, a birth mother is the biological mother. But if challenged on the grounds of genetics, DNA wins. I grew more and more upset, reading opinion after opinion that said I was indeed nothing to this child. I was an incubator, an oven. My feelings, my family, were meaningless. It wasn't that I was hoping to find an excuse to stake a claim to the baby. But I desperately wanted to read something that said I mattered.

Finally, I found some essays written by a Cornell law professor about our very predicament. Her opinion was the only one that recognized the value of my contribution to this life.

I didn't know whether to feel vindicated or abused. In fact, I felt both. There would be moments when I felt sweet pride at being the steward of a life. Then, in an instant, I would be slapped by the knowledge that my act of generosity was seen by the official world as irrelevant. My life mattered not at all, while at the same time this baby could not have a life without mine.

The next thing I knew, consumed with anger, I called Sean. Before he could get a word out, I started in.

"I can't do this. I don't want to give this gift. Why can't they give the gift? Why do we have to sacrifice? Why can't they sacrifice?"

"What are you trying to tell me?"

"I don't think I can go through with this. This is too much for me. Why can't the other family allow us to keep the baby?"

"Look, I'm coming home," Sean said.

"Don't. Stay at work. Coming home won't help," I said.

"I know this is so hard, but we will get through it together," Sean said.

I didn't know how I would get through this day, let alone the next eight months.

"I looked at all these opinions, all these different papers on the subject, and there is only one that says I matter," I continued.

"Carolyn, what does that matter, really? Our situation is unique."

"Yes, unique. That's a great word! Great! That doesn't mean that they can't use all these laws and decisions on me."

I must have sounded like a lunatic because Sean was speechless. I waited for a response from him, but there was only silence.

"Forget I called. Just forget it." And I hung up. I felt stupid for having a tantrum over the phone. I don't know what I was trying to accomplish, and in the end I think I just stressed Sean further.

As my emotions continued to flare, practical care was moving forward. That next day Dr. Read ordered an ultrasound much earlier than would have been done under normal conditions: exactly three weeks after the transfer. She wanted to know how many babies I was carrying. My blood work suggested a multiple pregnancy. We were scared to death that I was carrying triplets.

In the more than ten years I'd struggled with fertility, I'd spent a lot of time with Dr. Read's sonographer, Linda, who is a mini-celebrity among the doctor's patients. Whenever friends heard that Dr. Read was my obstetrician, they always commented, "Don't you love Linda?" The lights in her ultrasound room were dimmed, but she had decorated it with Christmas lights and a cheerful bulletin board tacked with pictures of babies from appreciative parents. Linda had an ease about her that made everyone smile. You couldn't help but greet her with a big hug, even if you knew when you entered her room that you might be facing bad news. Petite, graying, and fit, Linda was quick on her toes and had a witty sense of humor. Sometimes, when I'd fire rapid questions at her during an ultrasound, she would tell me, "Cool it, kiddo."

I held my breath while her internal ultrasound wand searched for evidence of the baby or babies. This ultrasound was so early, we knew there would be no heartbeat, only a gestational sac and a yolk. There were both, and only one of each. She searched my tubes to make sure there were no ectopics, and then we were finished. She printed a picture, handed it to me, and admitted that she didn't know what to say.

I grabbed the ultrasound image of the little one, and wondered, *Who are you?*

A few days later, Ryan was home sick, down with the bug that was traveling through our family. He was in the basement curled up with a blanket in front of the television. MK was getting whiny and needed a nap. I had just put her on the changing table and removed her diaper when I felt what I feared was a huge gush of blood. I instinctively crossed my legs and bent forward.

I got MK dressed quickly and laid her down haphazardly on the family room floor. I shuffled to the bathroom for some privacy, praying that I was wrong, but my worst fears were confirmed. I was bleeding.

"Damn. We hadn't even seen a heartbeat!"

I screamed for Ryan. He didn't respond at first, so I screamed louder. I think I scared him. He came flying up from the basement, and I asked for the phone so I could call Sean. Through the bathroom door, I directed him to pick MK up and put her up in her crib for her nap. I called Sean, whispering so that Ryan didn't hear me.

"I'm bleeding."

"What?"

"I'm bleeding. You need to come home."

"I'll be right there."

Afraid to move, I called Dr. Read from the bathroom. She told me to come in for another ultrasound.

I cleaned myself up as best I could and hobbled up the stairs to change my clothes. Once dressed, I lay down on the bed and waited. I feared I was losing someone else's baby. How would we explain this to the other family? They would blame me for this. Oh . . . and my fertility clinic. They'd be ecstatic. The loss of this baby would be a bullet dodged for them. My stomach flipped over with a wave of nausea. I didn't want to vomit, because I thought that would make me bleed more, so I willed it away.

I heard Sean come in through the door to the garage. *The force of raising my voice might hurt the baby,* I thought, so I lay quietly until he found me.

"Did you call the doctor?"

"Yes. We need to leave for an ultrasound. You need to wake MK, get her packed up and in her car seat. When that is all done, I'll get in the car."

I could hear MK crying as Sean woke her and bundled her up to go out in the cold. I felt bad for disrupting her nap. I felt bad for all of the disruptions. Mary Kate was growing and developing so rapidly as she neared her first birthday. I already recognized how distracted I'd become by this pregnancy, and I knew that she, Drew, and Ryan weren't getting the attention they deserved. But this time was crucial for MK. How was I going to concentrate on her milestones—first steps, first words—without thinking about how I wasn't going to get to see this baby pass those same milestones? I was so torn. Here was my precious daughter, the baby Sean and I had struggled for so long to have, and I was barely attending to some of the most important passages in her young life.

I carefully walked to the car and sat very still while we made our way to Dr. Read's office. It was a perfectly sunny day, and as we exited the highway to pull into her lot we fretted over what we were about to see. I thought of the ultrasound where we'd seen MK's dead twin in my uterus, then the horrid ultrasound in November 2006 when we were blindsided by the news that our baby had died in utero. I didn't want my body to fail another innocent life. I was petrified. Yet wouldn't a miscarriage be an escape? A way out? It didn't feel that way.

"This is probably the end," Sean said.

"I hope not," I replied.

"Me too," Sean said.

We were praying for this child, rooting for him or her with everything we had.

As the ultrasound image came up on the screen, I held my breath. I wanted to be the baby's biggest cheerleader and protector. So I prayed for the baby and for myself.

Please, God. Please don't let this baby die. Please, God, protect him or her. Let this baby grow to be healthy. Let this baby have a strong body and a stronger mind. Allow this baby to grow to know the joy of breathing and the opportunity to feel love. Please don't take this baby from me. Not now. Not before I can give the gift of life and I can receive that gift as well.

"Well, there you go. That's why you are bleeding."

Linda pointed to a big black blob underneath the gestational sac. I looked at Sean and shared with him the joy he reflected back to me. We both looked at the ultrasound screen again.

"Is that a subchorionic hematoma?"

In my hours and hours of reading about the science of pregnancy and what can go wrong, I had learned much about the conditions that cause a miscarriage. The subchorionic hematoma is a blood clot that forms, usually in the first trimester, and is far more common in

IVF pregnancies. My bleeding was the clot draining. The chances of a miscarriage because of a subchorionic were less than 2 percent. Linda continued searching.

"Uh . . . no heartbeat yet, but the baby has grown since Friday, and the gestational sac looks good. Everything is measuring right on target. Now the blood is sitting on your cervix, so you are probably going to have more bleeding."

She captured a bunch of images and escorted us to an examining room to meet with Dr. Read, who said the blood would either drain or reabsorb. Though Dr. Read was confident that the clot would not harm the baby, I asked for another blood test so we could confirm that my pregnancy hormones—the HCG reading—were continuing to rise. I knew that a fetal heartbeat would be detectable at 5,000. I wanted to double-check that the jig wasn't already up.

Dr. Read agreed and handed me a lab slip. We scheduled another ultrasound in four days, and Linda shared with us that if there was no heartbeat by then, there would be reason for concern. Dr. Read said to take it easy until then—lifting MK was fine, but nothing more strenuous.

On the car ride home, I fretted about what the boys would think. My guess was that they were already suspicious. Poor Ryan heard me screaming in the bathroom for the phone, then Sean arrived in the middle of the day. Next thing he knew, we were scurrying out the door. Ryan asked where we were going, but we didn't answer. He asked again . . . still no answer. Then he said, "Never mind." How was I supposed to pretend that everything was fine when I was lying in bed all day?

The next day, when I had to drive to the lab for blood work, I knew that, even as light as she was, I should put MK in the stroller and wheel her into the lab. I was feeling weak and woozy from all the blood loss, but I had to continue to be a mom, to run the house and provide the meals. I was trying to figure out what we needed for dinner as I pulled into the pharmacy drive-thru to retrieve prescriptions. When it was my turn at the window, I reached back for my purse. Where was it? I twisted around to check the backseat, but it wasn't there. I'd left my purse at the lab. "Sweet mother of God, can I catch a break, please?" I screamed in my car. I caught the startled look of the pharmacist, who I'm pretty sure was glad that there was a pane of bulletproof glass between us.

After I got my purse and returned for the prescriptions, I had to pick up Drew early from school for an orthodontist appointment. While he was at the doctor, I shuffled through the market like I was eighty years old. I figured keeping my legs together would prevent the baby from falling out. After the appointment, Drew wasn't feeling well, so I took him home instead of back to school. There I got a call from Dr. Read's office saying my blood work was good. I lay down that afternoon in hopes of resting while Mary Kate napped.

Sleep had been elusive since we learned of the mistake. I needed to get to a point where the situation wasn't consuming my thoughts every minute of the day. I prayed for the strength to move past my anger toward the person in the laboratory who made the mistake. I knew I had a right to be angry, but I didn't want to walk around being mad all day. How could I forgive this person? Did I have to forgive him or her? Was that the only way I would get some peace?

Focus on the baby, I thought. We'd just dodged a tragedy. The baby was strong, and I was strong enough to survive this.

SEAN

THAT NIGHT I COULDN'T SLEEP, and I saw that Carolyn was restless too. It seemed silly to pretend that either of us was sleeping when we both were so shaken. I touched her on the shoulder, and she opened her eyes immediately.

"Carolyn, that drive to the ultrasound was terrifying," I said. "I can't imagine what it was like for you. The fear of losing the baby is still with me."

"I know," she said as she turned to face me. "With all the problems we've had lately, it surprised me how much I love this child already."

"The baby is already part of our family," I said.

As we lay in bed I started to understand that the child inside of Carolyn was now someone I needed to protect. How long he or she would be with us was already defined by law and by the choices we made, but for these eight months I was the baby's father. After that, Carolyn and I would want to be a part of the baby's life, but it would never be the same kind of connection we were going to have for these few months. Although I never could fully comprehend what Carolyn was going through, I could support her by taking on the planning and organizing needed to set up a structure that would guide us throughout the pregnancy. And that was a task that played to my strengths.

Ever since I was young, I have been someone who likes to plan out everything. My parents taught me the importance of planning, and I went into a profession where I help individuals and families plan for their futures. My own financial planning began at age five when my mom drove me to the bank to open a savings account in my name. When I had earned enough money for a deposit, I loved watching the teller make another entry in my ledger book and seeing my balance increase. Heck, I do not think I took a withdrawal out of that bank account until I paid a college tuition bill.

After our sessions with Kevin Anderson and the one with Father Cardone the day we found out about the pregnancy, I had written down several lists of action items. When I went for my run, they were just in my head. The next morning, after my talk with Carolyn, I woke up early so I would have time to write down everything that this mistake had introduced into our lives.

I began with the fundamental choices we made to (1) continue the pregnancy and (2) not fight for custody. All of our problems and plans flowed from these two decisions. Next, I wrote down the tasks and difficulties that resulted from those two decisions and divided them into categories. When they became so numerous that they crowded the edge of the page, a light went on in my head. We needed a binder. I had to smile at that. There are few problems that can't be solved with a big black binder.

As an adult, my ledger became my binders. I have binders for work, for all of the teams I coach, and for our own financial plans and estate planning. I got one of the black "mega" binders out of the box I keep in the basement. As with all of my binders, the new one needed a name to capture the essence of the situation. After some deliberation, I titled it "The Sean and Carolyn Savage CF File." (If anyone asked, I decided I'd tell them CF stood for "Caring Family.") Inside the binder I made a table of contents on a page entitled "Sean and Carolyn Savage: The Road Never Traveled." I labeled the headings with letters A through Z, guessing that I'd be adding more categories in the next eight months.

a. Information from Clinic or Legal Representatives
b. Prioritization Categories and Timeline: The Lists
c. Family Law Information
d. Genetic Family Information and Communication
e. Communication Planning to Family and Friends
f. Savage Family Security Plan
g. Other Legal Issues
h. Expenses Incurred (Direct and Indirect)
i. Catholic Church Information
j. Medical Documentation: Ultrasound Pictures/Medical Records

For me the stiff dividers between the categories illustrated the structure that would support my view of the crisis and where it might lead. These eight months could bury us under paper if I let them. I also got out the box of plastic sleeves I use to file documents. I knew from experience that, with plastic sleeves, if we had a question about one of our decisions or about what one of the other parties involved had said, we'd be able to get our hands on the answer in seconds. Slipping the handful of documents we'd already produced into the plastic made me feel as though we were starting to get a handle on the situation.

Then I devised another category—"Beyond the Stuff"—to cover the core emotional items, including:

- Open discussion of thoughts and feelings
- No judgment
- Discussions twice a week on personal impact
- Control anxiety and limit turning into opponents of each other

These last categories were the most important because they would support our psychological well-being.

As the Friday ultrasound appointment approached, I comforted myself with the reminder that we were doing all we could. Either there would be a heartbeat or the pregnancy was over. We would be capable of dealing with either of those outcomes.

At Dr. Read's, Carolyn handed Mary Kate to me right away, and together we walked into the ultrasound room. Linda was in a good mood, as always, remarking on how cute MK's outfit was and ready with a quip about the crappy weather. Carolyn assumed her position on the ultrasound table, while I sat next to her, gripping MK like a security blanket. Carolyn closed her eyes as Linda prepped her for the ultrasound.

As Linda turned on the screen and grabbed the wand, I know Carolyn was saying a little prayer for the baby and for us. It couldn't have been more than a few seconds, when Linda said, "Well, guys, we have a ticker."

"Thank God," Carolyn whispered. The baby's heartbeat was a mere ninety-five beats per minute.

"Is that normal?" Carolyn asked.

"Yes, it probably just started beating this morning," Linda said.

Carolyn and I smiled for the first time since the day we received the news. When I saw the heartbeat, the pregnancy went from an intangible to an absolute. We just watched this child's heart start to beat. In a few weeks, he or she would have legs, feet, arms, fingers, and toes, all because of Carolyn. This was real. This was life. At this point, the thought of giving up this baby seemed inconceivable.

As we walked out, Carolyn was beaming. She said, "A heart holds a person's soul. It allows one to love, and to be loved." Love feeds the heart, and now this baby's was growing. I think it was at that very moment that this little person burrowed into our hearts forever.

CHAPTER 6

One Step Forward, Two Steps Back

Our lawyer sent this note to the genetic parents' lawyer on March 11, 2009.

> *Attached please find an ultrasound taken on this date. My clients would like your clients to know that as of March 11, 2009, the baby was measuring 7w1d and had a heart rate of 129 beats per minute indicating continued healthy development. Their next appointment and ultrasound is scheduled for Tuesday, March 24, 2009. If anything develops with the pregnancy before then, they will communicate that through my office.*
>
> *At this early stage, my clients are not comfortable agreeing to further communication. They will continue to provide updates regarding medical progress after appointments. They will also communicate any other developments that arise regarding the health and development of the pregnancy.*
>
> *My clients do request that your clients understand how devastated they are by this situation. Their journey to expanding their family has consumed the past twelve years of their lives and has included a lot of loss and heartbreak along the way. They are still in shock regarding this situation and are fraught with anxiety regarding the long-lasting*

ramifications that this situation will have on their family and lives.
They are simply trying to cope with their grief at this early stage.

They do understand how anxiety ridden your clients must be
regarding the health of their unborn child. The only thing they can
communicate to ease your clients' fears is that they will treat this unborn
child as if it was their own. They have superb medical care and are fol-
lowing the advice of their physician.

Lastly, my clients have agreed to receive a list of questions that your
clients may have for them. Please forward the list to me as soon as your
clients have it completed.

Respectfully Yours,
Mary E. Smith

CAROLYN

I HAD NEVER FELT so stifled in my life. At a moment when I needed
support more than anything, I wasn't allowed to share my burden
with my friends and my family. The only people I could talk to
about my heartbreak were Sean, the lawyers, and Kevin Anderson,
thank goodness. All of them were in agreement that I should say
nothing. I had never lived in such an interior world. At the same
time, I'd never had so much to say.

My mom and I chat on the phone several times a week. Besides
the family gossip, I know her thought process about every decision
she's made to redecorate the house. I also know, before the guests
arrive, the menu of every dinner party she's ever had. After she's
filled me in, she wants to know everything about me. We talk about
the kids first. At some point in the conversation, I put her on speaker
to sing to MK. My mom doesn't have what you would call an ear for
music, but she loves to sing, and MK loves it too.

Since we found out about the pregnancy, each time I talked

with my mom on the phone, right before I hung up, I wanted to say, "Wait, wait . . . help me . . . please," but I never did. We would tell them as soon as Dr. Read deemed the pregnancy viable. I was counting the weeks until then. Meanwhile, on our winter vacation, we were walking into a situation that would test my ability to keep my mouth shut.

Shortly after the lawyer sent that letter to the other family, we were scheduled to make our annual visit to Cape Coral, Florida, where my parents spend the winter. While we love visiting my parents, we have always been sensitive about not crowding them in the modest place they rent, so we rent a condo on nearby Sanibel Island. That way, we can see them as much as we want but not cramp their style. After Dr. Read cleared me to travel, I tried to visualize visiting my mom and not breathing a word of what was going on inside of me. It would be sort of like being a teenager all over again, minus the door slamming.

I knew this trip would be tough because it wasn't just my mom who would have her eyes on me but also the Corey family, my parents' best friends since I was a small child. When I was young, my family spent weekends on our sailboat in Sarnia, Canada. Among the few constants on those weekends was knowing that if there was wind, we would be under sail. The second was that, if we were under sail, we were racing the Coreys. Their boat was docked three slips down from ours, and they had three kids around the same ages as my brothers and me. Tip and Jean Corey were also going to be in Cape Coral during our vacation.

The Coreys might provide enough of a social life for most women, but not my mom, a woman who can make friends absolutely anywhere she goes. We have often joked that if my mom were ever incarcerated, she'd have a gourmet group, a book club, and a garden club up and off the ground within her first few days in the clink. Over the winters my parents have spent at Cape Coral, she's increased her circle of friends well beyond the Coreys. As Sean and the boys packed the car for our drive to the airport, I was hoping that Jean and my mom, or any of the many other people in Cape Coral who have seen us over the years, would be unable to pick up anything different about Sean and me on this visit.

When we arrived in Florida, the weather was heavenly. Every day after sleeping in, I would venture down to the pool to soak in the glorious sunshine as I sat on the steps and splashed around with Mary Kate. The condo resort had some seasonal residents who met daily under the awning at the pool. I enjoyed eavesdropping as they discussed the new manicurist or some woman's botched hairdo. They were also pretty opinionated on the subject of whatever current event had usurped the television talk shows the night before. I wished that was the most important thing on my mind.

One morning, while I was sitting on the steps of the pool playing with MK, one of the "awning ladies" swam over to talk.

"So, what do you think about that lady who had eight babies?"

I paused for a moment, trying to figure out the right way to respond to a question about Nadya Suleman. I suddenly realized that I took observations about the "OctoMom" personally.

"I think she was under the care of an incredibly irresponsible fertility doctor."

"What do you mean?"

"Well, 85 percent of women who get pregnant using IVF give birth to a single baby. Ten percent have twins, and the other 5 percent may end up with triplets or more, but octuplets? The doctor who thought it was ethical to transfer six embryos into a woman in her thirties who already had six children should lose his medical license."

She thought about this for a moment, while doing her water aerobics.

"I've never heard of a woman using IVF and only getting one baby," she said.

I held up MK.

"Well, she's an IVF baby, and we only had one."

I was a little annoyed, but I knew that her misinformed opinion about the likelihood of multiple births with IVF was common.

She commented on what a beautiful baby MK was, and then bounced away from me, sensing that she had struck a nerve.

I watched her climb out of the pool, and head back to her friends under the awning. I knew I was getting talked about, since they were all suddenly trying not to stare at me. I imagined what she was saying: "You see that mom down there with that baby. That baby is an IVF baby, and she only had one. Can you believe that?" I thought to myself, *Oh, woman, if you only knew.*

And if she knew that this time next year, she might be hearing our story in the news, would she treat me differently?

What if I had been free to tell anyone I chose what was really happening? Maybe that woman at the pool wouldn't have looked at me with such wide eyes, as if MK were some kind of medical curiosity. She might have hugged me and told me what a good thing I was doing. That's what I wanted from my mom and dad. I wanted them to be able to hold me in their arms the way I held Drew, Ryan, and Mary Kate. I wanted them to tell me that it was going to be all right, that they were there, and that they too would make sure no harm came to me or my baby.

I saw my mom and dad every day, and I was grateful that those occasions were busy. If it was dinner at my mom's, she was the demon of the kitchen producing one incredible meal after the other. When we went out with the kids in the afternoons, the kids took center stage. I was relieved when we'd made it all the way to Wednesday without Mom and me getting a chance to have some time alone.

With no girlfriends to chat with, and the pregnancy taking up most of my energy, my thoughts often drifted to the genetic mom. I thought about how worried she would be if she knew what had happened when we thought we'd lost the baby. What if she had been trying for years to have a child and this was the first success, but the pregnancy was in some other woman? I bet her mind was whirling too. Maybe it was good that we couldn't communicate with each other right then. Who knows what we would have said?

On Wednesday we were all eating lunch in the condo when I heard the *ping* of a delivered e-mail on my computer. I opened it immediately and found a message from our lawyer informing us that she had attached a letter from the genetic family. I hesitated before reading it, as Mary had included a warning. "Think carefully before reading this, Carolyn." Was she worried that it could be hurtful?

Do I really want to hear what they have to say? Of course I do. Plus, we already explained to them how upset we are. We invited them to send us a list of questions, so surely that is all this is. I should read it.

I took a deep breath, opened the attachment, and read the letter quickly. As my eyes scanned the three-page letter, I realized, to my surprise, that this letter was much more than a list of questions.

Wait! I'm not ready for this. This is too much.

My gut was telling me to stop reading, but my eyes couldn't help but pour over the information that the genetic mother of my baby provided.

After reading it once I was in shock. My heart was racing, my arms and legs were numb, and I was shaking. *Calm down, Carolyn. It's okay. You read it too fast. Read it again. Surely, you are misunderstanding something.*

I read the letter again, searching for something that I felt wasn't there. I desperately wanted to read that she felt terrible for us, that she couldn't imagine our despair, that they'd do whatever they could to help us. As I reviewed each sentence, the sentiments of the letter were slamming into me like bullets piercing my heart. Those thoughts, those feelings that I wanted to hear were surprisingly absent.

I must have been visibly upset because, before I knew it, Sean was at my side, reading over my shoulder.

Read it again and read it carefully. The messages you long to hear are there! You are just missing them.

I started over at the beginning, but after reading the letter a third time, I was exasperated.

"I can't believe this!" I blurted out. "This woman sent me a laundry list as to why this is so horrible for her. My God, they are getting a baby out of this."

"Hold on, Carolyn. I have to read it again."

"Sean, you can read this letter a hundred times and it won't change the fact that it's heartless."

Sean studied the words on the page, but my anger boiled over. I grabbed my sunglasses, stomped out to the beach, and took a seat at the water's edge.

I reviewed the letter in my head. I had invited them to send us a list of questions. Instead, the genetic mother, Shannon, sent a letter telling me about how she was going to lose her privacy, how Shannon was going to have to explain this to her co-workers, and how Shannon thought she might have gotten three babies if the embryos had been transferred to her womb. And worst of all, Shannon decided that God did this. "God for some reason decided that another woman would carry this baby for me." That stung worst of all. Where exactly did Shannon think that left me and my family in God's eyes?

As I dug my toes into the sand, I tried to shake off the first impression this letter gave me. How could she have written me such a self-focused letter? Was she trying to convince me that she had it worse? And if she was, what does that say about her ability to show compassion to us as this situation unfolds? I shut my eyes and took a few calming breaths. *Carolyn, slow down!* I told myself. *Try to understand where Shannon was coming from when she wrote the letter.*

I tried to imagine how frightened Shannon was about not knowing who we were. I'm betting she was trying to encourage us to reveal ourselves so she could know more about the situation. Unfortunately, her strategy backfired because the letter placed a fear in my heart that had not existed before. Could her sentiments be proof that what we were doing to give them a baby did not really matter that much? Could she be saying that once the baby was in their arms, their first goal would be to erase everything we had done in order to claim this child as truly their own? I shivered at the thought of us being removed from the equation of this child's life. I had spent a lot of time trying to convince myself that after I delivered this baby, we would mercifully be given the opportunity to know him or her forever. Now I wasn't so sure.

SEAN

OUT OF THE CORNER of my eye, I could see Carolyn's mood changing as she read. She was shifting in her chair as she got more and more angry.

I wondered what she could be reading that was upsetting her so much, so I went over to the computer and started reading over her shoulder. As I read, she got up and paced back and forth. I was surprised at the inward focus of the woman who wrote it, but tried not to take too much offense. I knew it was normal for people to spend almost all of the time thinking about themselves. I cut Shannon some slack because she did not know us. She did write that she appreciated that we were continuing the pregnancy.

Carolyn was searching the letter for something that wasn't there. Simple sentences on the page were like blows to her heart. She was so vulnerable then, tired, distraught, and not herself. My goal in Sanibel was to take care of everything for Carolyn in the hopes that rest and relaxation would soothe some of her anxiety. I took the early shift with Mary Kate and kept the boys out of the condo once Carolyn was up. When she and MK napped, I tended to do stuff from work. I hoped that, if I kept to this schedule, Carolyn could get more than ten hours of sleep a night and a lot of rest during the day. I knew a healthy mom helped make for a happy baby, and I wanted to support both.

Perfect. Well, not really. The trip brought Carolyn and me in close proximity for twenty-four hours a day, but we were hardly close. If she wasn't sleeping, she was there with us but somehow far away, her mind lost in some other space where she was trying to comprehend what was happening to her. I missed her. And rest alone was not enough to calm her.

"C'mon, Carolyn, let's give them the benefit of the doubt for now," I said.

"She's not thankful to me, Sean. She thinks I'm her surrogate!" Carolyn said. "She can only think about how hard this all is for her."

"She said she was grateful," I said. "They don't even know us."

"She didn't say she was grateful, she expressed her gratitude," Carolyn said. "Passive voice, like she's saying it against her will. I hate this letter."

"Hate the letter?" I was surprised. "Carolyn, you are not a hater! What you are doing is beautiful, a beautiful expression of your love of life. When they understand everything we are doing for them, they will love and admire you."

"That doesn't mean I have to love everybody," Carolyn said. "Everybody around is sure they know what I should and shouldn't do, even how I should feel. This is what happens when someone as deeply flawed as me tries to do the right thing. There are many moments when I'm not feeling the way I'm supposed to feel, but I'm trying to do the right thing anyway."

"Carolyn, once this other couple knows our story and understands the depths of our despair, they will be so thankful that they will do what they can to help us. I could not imagine the other family would intentionally want to make things worse."

"Well, they have!" she said, and she stomped out of the condo to take a walk on the beach.

Embers were smoldering between us, and the conditions were ripe for a fire to break out. It did not help that Carolyn was turning forty that week, an emotional milestone in the best of times. Carolyn's mom was planning a big party for her fortieth birthday. Linda was so involved in preparations for the party that she didn't observe anything different about Carolyn. Carolyn's brother Mike, his wife, Jenny, and their three boys were beginning their vacation that weekend, and Mr. and Mrs. Corey and their oldest son, Stephen, and his family were also there. Normally, we would have been happy to celebrate with them, but neither Carolyn nor I was looking forward to this get-together.

The night of Carolyn's birthday party we enjoyed the usual "Linda Spread" of great food, and Carolyn's dad was busy at the blender making his signature drink, "Byron Blasters." We knew that they would be suspicious if Carolyn didn't slurp down a few of her dad's rum-drenched concoctions, but we had a plan. Earlier that morning, Carolyn had bought some green apple wine coolers (her favorites), removed the bottle caps, emptied the contents, and funneled Sprite into each bottle. Then she screwed the lids back on and brought them to the party as her undercover beverages for the night.

There were twenty-five guests that night, and coincidentally, about half of them also had a birthday in March. Instead of decorating the cake in just Carolyn's honor, Linda had everyone's names on it. When it was time to blow out the candles, Linda, who had enjoyed a few blasters that evening, decided there would be a roll call of all the guests with March birthdays. Everyone had to say their age and shout out a signature cheer. She started with the oldest, so Carolyn wasn't first. Mr. Corey started by declaring his eightieth birthday and then giving us his famous "woop woop."

As the older guests continued exclaiming their ages and something that they were proud of, I saw Carolyn frantically searching her mind for something to say other than, "I'm Carolyn, I'm forty and knocked up with the wrong baby!"

I caught her eye as her turn grew closer, and I knew she could see the empathy on my face. Before I knew it, she blurted out, "I'm Carolyn, I'm forty, and I'm fabulous!"

Everyone cheered, and we smiled, but she told me later that she just wanted to disappear. Not only had she just enthusiastically employed one of the cheesiest clichés known to man, but she knew deep down that there was nothing fabulous going on.

CAROLYN

THE MORNING AFTER the big birthday bash, I sat curled up on a lounge chair on the balcony of our condo thinking about this child's genetic mother, Shannon, and the baby's genetic father, Paul. For weeks, I had longed to know whose child I was carrying. I wanted to respect and admire the people to whom we were giving this gift. Instead, my introduction to them was a letter that troubled me in ways I never expected. I looked out at the sea, hugging my knees to my chest, trying very hard not to cry. Was I overreacting? I reached over for the laptop and started to read the letter again.

Sean's comments from the day before were still with me: "Honey, I know the letter upset you, but I'm not sure what you expected."

I don't know what I expected either. I guess I had convinced myself that the mother of this child was worse off than us regarding her infertility struggles and that bearing this child and giving the baby to them would be the answer to their prayers. But Shannon wrote that they did one IVF. Only one, and got twins. And now she is getting a third child from the one IVF. Rarely do couples get an entire family from one IVF. She didn't seem to understand how lucky she was!

In fact, it was clear from the letter that she felt extremely un-lucky as she went on to complain about how "stressful" this was for her. She also said she felt "powerless"! I understood why, but I wondered if she understood that I had lost power over my body. To make matters worse, she went on to imply that if the three embryos had been transferred into her uterus instead of mine, she'd have given birth to three babies. Like somehow my body killed some of her babies. I reread that paragraph just to make sure I was not mistaken

> We were told that three embryos survived the thawing, but they didn't look good. We were thrilled to learn that one had survived. Though, I wonder "what if" I had been implanted with three, would more than one have survived?

Sean was astonished when he reread that portion of the letter. He thought that remark may have been the most upsetting, but he thought there was a close second. It was when Shannon wrote

> With a newborn, I'd have to take time off from work. I really don't want my co-workers knowing about my personal business. So, I've thought about just taking a medical leave vs. a maternity leave. I could say that I have adopted a baby, but that wouldn't be right. I've thought about saying nothing and that it was a "miracle."

I agreed with Sean that this portion of the letter was perplexing. It just didn't seem appropriate to complain to us about the sudden appearance of a newborn when we were being faced with explaining the sudden loss of a newborn. I guess she's in a tough spot, though, as she included a statement saying they didn't tell people they used IVF for her twins, which raised another concern. I understand the desire to keep your reproductive life private, but dishonesty is never a good way to go. And, based on her statements, it looks like she was considering hiding where this baby was coming from. Could this mean that there will be a conflict over whether we tell the truth about this mess? Sean and I are certainly not willing to lie about any of this!

I had desperately wanted Shannon to say "thank you" for what we were doing. And the words "thank you" did appear, yet the sentence where she imparts that sentiment contained a trap for me. I read it again.

Thank you for continuing the pregnancy and treating it as if it were your own.

She did say "thank you," but this pregnancy is my own. Could this mean that she thinks it is her pregnancy in my body? Like I hijacked her baby or something?

I looked up from my laptop, growing more and more frustrated with the letter and the stress it was causing me. I knew I needed to have an open mind about Shannon. She was in pain too, but there were many sentiments in the letter that hurt. I had spent the last five weeks feeling sorry for her, and I assumed that she'd be overwhelmed with empathy for our situation. Unfortunately, when I read the letter, I didn't feel empathy. I felt insensitivity, and if she is insensitive now, I was scared of how she could treat us when the baby is born, or after.

I was relieved to learn that this baby would be raised by a committed couple. Shannon and her husband, Paul, had been married for seven years. And this child would have two older sisters who I am sure will adore him, so that was great news. However, I was struck at what was missing at the end of the letter. Paul's signature. Just Shannon signed it, and I wondered what that meant.

I knew I needed to stop analyzing the letter. It was raising more questions and causing more stress and anger than I could handle. Maybe she was just trying to commiserate with me about the whole situation and she just got carried away with her complaints. I needed to adopt Sean's take on the whole thing. He said we should hope for the best and proceed cautiously with Shannon.

To try to find a release for my anger I decided to do the one thing I thought would help: write Shannon a response. I knew I'd never send it, so I opened the vents and said anything and everything in an attempt to unburden my heart.

Letter to Shannon (never sent)

Dear Shannon,

I'm not sure what I'm supposed to say to you. When I read your letter I was surprised by how focused you were on the problems that you were facing surrounding this ridiculous situation. My husband asked me if there was anything that you could have written that wouldn't have upset me. I think he was surprised to hear that my answer was yes. I think a simple note expressing your incredible gratitude would have been sufficient. In addition, an acknowledgment of how unbelievably awful our situation is, and how you are praying for us would have been nice. I wasn't prepared to hear you compare our situations as equal. And I surely wasn't prepared to listen to all of your reasons that this is so awful for you. It was like you wanted to go toe to toe about who had it worse. Well . . . if that is what you want, here you go.

It is unfortunate that you may have to "out" yourself regarding the use of IVF and the facts surrounding the conception of your twin girls. That information should have been able to remain private. Since you chose, for personal reasons, to lead others to believe that your twins were conceived "naturally," (which I have to say is a term I take great offense to, as it deems IVF children to be what . . . unnatural?) I can see how it might be awkward to admit that you misled others to believe that you had just been surprisingly "blessed."

As for you struggling to explain this to your 8th-grade students and your teaching colleagues, we have similar but more staggering dilemmas here. Imagine trying to explain to your twelve- and fourteen-year-old sons that mom is pregnant but has to give the baby away in the delivery room because the baby isn't hers. Imagine the horror of having to listen to your PARENTS explain what IVF is, and how their sister was conceived. Then imagine them having to explain this to their friends.

Of course, this will require explanations to absolutely everyone who is part of our lives. After all, we can't hide a pregnancy. Everyone knows what we went through to get our daughter. Everyone knows how devoted we are to our children and family. No one would believe that we gave a baby up for adoption, and we would never collude to allow anyone to think that we had another baby die on us. We have no choice but to tell the truth, and the news will spread like wildfire. People we have never met before are going to know our private reproductive business. The thought of this makes me physically ill.

You made many assumptions in your letter about me having a positive experience during this situation. You also assumed that I'd be able to just pick up afterward and go on to have my own child. Please let me explain a few things about the long-term effects that this situation is having on my ability to do just that. I just turned forty. Do you have any idea what that does to my chances of having a successful go at my own embryos? At the very earliest, I'll be forty-one and a half by the time I'm able to attempt a transfer with my own embryos. At forty, my chances for success plummeted and every passing year after forty drops my chances further. Our goal was to get after our own embryos before I turned forty to increase our chances for success. We had hoped to provide our daughter with a sibling that was close in age to her. It was important to me, especially after losing her twin. Now, all of that has been jeopardized.

I'm sorry that you are haunted with "what ifs" surrounding this situation. Trust me, I couldn't agree more that your embryos do not belong in my uterus. In fact, there were other women having transfers on February 6th and I can confidently say that your embryos would have been better off being transferred into any of them. You see, I haven't carried a baby to term since 1994. Your baby will be my third C-section. The risks with a fourth C-section are significant. This situation has left me beyond screwed.

The hardest thing about this is the mental torture that I put myself through regarding having to let this baby go. He is in me. I've been praying for this baby long before we knew he was coming. He will give me heartburn, varicose veins, stretch marks, and tears at the dumbest things. I am crabby with my husband, and intimacy is off-limits for the duration. The idea that I have to go through all of that, and then hand the baby off to someone else in the delivery room is too much for me. We know we are doing the right thing. We know this is not your fault. It is just so hard.

I believe in God. I have a strong and devoted faith life. I do not believe that God sits up in heaven and decides who gets to struggle with cancer, and who gets to struggle with infertility, and who gets this tragedy and that blessing. I believe in random acts that affect people's lives. I believe that my faith guides me in how to deal with the events that present themselves in my life. This event is giving me a challenge. I am searching for grace, and it's hard to find right now.

I hate you sometimes. I hate you for wanting this child and assuming that we will happily hand it over. I hate you for assuming that this will be easy because it is not a twin pregnancy. I hate you for assuming that our situations are the same. They are so different. A year from now you will be cuddling your new baby. We, on the other hand, will be dealing with the wreckage left in the aftermath of this disaster. Still waiting, and wondering if we have a chance for our dream and wondering if there is any hope left. I especially hate you for insinuating that God did this. That God decided that this would happen and that "another woman would carry this baby for you." Do you think God thinks I deserve this? Do you think God decided to put my family through this? There is no way God did this. God would not have chosen me. I am not strong enough. I am not loving enough. I am not patient enough. No, God did not do this. In fact, I'm pretty sure an inexcusably distracted medical professional did this . . . not God.

I am just so scared. I am scared that you think I am nothing and that I am undeserving of your sensitivity and respect. I am afraid that you will hurt me, take this child, and leave me with nothing. I am scared of losing this baby. I already love him. I will always love him. I hope you understand that.

I know I will never send this letter. I know you don't deserve my anger, my ugliness, or my hatred. So it is better right now for me to say nothing, and pray for strength, patience, and love, because the only way I think I can survive this is to learn to like you. I need to be happy for you and your family. I truly don't know if I have that in me and a lot of this will depend on you. I guess time will tell.

Carolyn

I finished writing, reviewed what I wrote, and was ashamed. I knew I was being irrational and harsh, but as I reread my letter, over and over again, I knew it captured my anguish. And I felt better just getting it down on paper.

I flipped my laptop closed and prayed to God for help.

Please, God, help me be stronger. Help me find the strength I need to accept this situation. Help me endure this suffering with grace, and help me understand why this happened. Please, God, help me. Please.

CHAPTER 7

Keeping the Secret

CAROLYN

THE NIGHT WE GOT HOME from Florida, I did something dumb. I read Shannon's letter again. I don't know why I felt I needed to do it. I was in bed thinking about the letter and the baby, and I started to cry. Was she that insensitive to the suffering we were enduring? If she was, how would she behave at the dreaded delivery? I imagined her jumping up and down when my baby was handed to her. She would celebrate our grief, our tragedy, our sadness, as her joy, her triumph, her miracle. Even though I knew we would have taken our baby from her if the situation had been reversed, I resented her as if she were the one who had done this to us.

I tried to cry quietly so Sean wouldn't hear. I didn't want to upset him. He couldn't help me anyway. Despite my efforts, he woke up to my tears.

"What's wrong?"

I didn't want to answer.

"What's wrong?" he persisted.

His questions made my tears come quicker. I really wanted my bed to open up and swallow me. I finally answered.

"How am I going to do this? I think God screwed up."

I turned to face him, but his back was to me. I waited for him to turn around, but he didn't.

"How can God think that I can do this?"

Still no response.

My body shook with sobs, yet he hadn't rolled over. As I waited, I began to feel that, by keeping his back turned to me, he was scolding me for being upset. This made it worse.

"I want this baby. He feels like mine. I can't give him away."

Sean's silence only upset me further.

I finally went into the bathroom and closed the door behind me. I leaned my back against the wall and slid down to the floor, burying my head in my knees. If I couldn't speak to Sean about this, where would I turn? I was struggling with the insinuation that this was all part of God's plan. The few people who knew of my pregnancy had said that when they heard the news. Really? God planned this? Not the gentle, loving, and constant God I worshiped. The idea that all of this had happened because of God made me angrier than I had ever been. It also made me feel helpless and out of control. I prayed to God.

Where the hell are you in this? This is your plan? What did I do to deserve this? I have been a good woman. I have sacrificed for you. I dedicated my career to you. This is how you repay me? You force suffering on me that I cannot bear? I don't think I can be pregnant and deliver a baby to another woman. How will I withstand watching her celebrate my sorrow? You chose the wrong woman. I am not strong enough.

I begged God for strength and for courage, but both eluded me. I felt like I was such a wreck all the time. My world, once so open and alive with many friends and all of my commitments to the boys and to the community, had shrunk to the square footage of our bedroom. My mood was terrible too. I am the kind of person who tries to think the best of others and always give them the benefit of the doubt, but this event had changed that. I imagined that Sean was disappointed in me for saying such hateful things and that he was annoyed with me for being sick, having no energy, being so crabby, and having to struggle to stay positive even in the happy moments.

Please make me stronger. Please make me a better person. If you can't, then just let me die.

This thought immediately conjured guilt in my heart. I would never want to leave my kids. I would never wish that kind of tragedy into their lives.

I was so upset by my mind lurching between such extreme feelings that I felt nauseous. I steadied myself against the bathroom door, hoping that having something firm against my back would keep my stomach from spinning. It didn't. I bent over the toilet, throwing up, trying like hell to stop the retching because I feared it might hurt the baby. Finally it subsided, and I rested my head on the toilet seat and tried to catch my breath. *Calm down, Carolyn. Calm down.* I shuffled over to the sink to brush my teeth and wash my face. What I saw in the mirror was pitiful. I was pale, my eyes were again bloodshot from crying, and my neck and face were covered in splotches. I knew I needed to get some sleep, but I wondered what the heck Sean was doing in turning his back to me. Wasn't he worried about me? Didn't he care?

I finally turned out the light and went into the bedroom. I couldn't see anything, but I knew Sean had not moved. I turned my back to him, stared at the window hoping for sleep to come. I apologized to God and closed my eyes, feeling alone and ashamed.

SEAN

I WOKE UP MONDAY morning feeling guilty for having abandoned Carolyn the night before. I knew she was hurting, but I was hurting as well, and so exhausted. Sunday I had woken early to take the kids to mass while Carolyn rested. There I prayed for peace and the strength to keep going. I kept the kids busy all day as I did household chores. When my head hit the pillow Sunday night, my service-to-others gas tank was empty. I drifted to sleep while Carolyn was crying. No excuse.

I missed the easy way we used to be with each other, our private jokes and that hour I treasured just before we fell asleep at night. We hadn't been intimate in more than two months because of her medical status, and it seemed that as each day passed things got worse at home and between us. As the distance grew, my natural reaction was to shut down. Tunnel vision helped me avoid escalating the tension between us. We didn't need to fight. Fighting would only make things worse, and I did not want to add more trouble to our life. In the meantime, I had to slough off the pain of it and just get through.

The boys were starting to get suspicious. Sunday afternoon I was in my chair in the family room jotting down my weekly list of tasks: those for the next day and longer goals for the rest of that week. The house was serene. Carolyn was napping, and so was Mary Kate. Drew entered the family room and stood next to my chair. I looked up into his serious young face.

"Dad, Mom is always in bed lately. What's wrong with her?"

His question broke my heart.

"Mom hasn't been feeling well, but it's not serious, and she's going to be just fine."

Drew nodded his head and left the room.

I hope I comforted him. Were we really shielding the children from this trauma by keeping the secret? The tentacles of the problem seemed to grasp at every corner of our lives.

Right before walking out of our bedroom Monday morning to go to work, I stroked Carolyn's hair while she was waking up. "I am sorry for ignoring you last night. It was wrong, and I should have been there to help you. I have no excuse. I'll pick you up for the ultrasound today if you would rather not drive."

She smiled sleepily. "I'll call the doctor's office to schedule a time and call you. I love you very much. Have a good day at work," she said.

"I love you and will see you later."

The week after that ultrasound we were officially in week ten of the pregnancy, and we celebrated Carolyn's fortieth birthday with friends. While Carolyn didn't feel much like celebrating, all of her girlfriends had huge blowouts on their big day. If she didn't have one they might think something was wrong at home. I was happy she agreed to allow me to treat her and her girlfriends to dinner in a private room of a nice restaurant, while the guys watched NCAA basketball games at our house, awaiting the women's return for cake and cocktails.

On the Friday of the party, I left work early and stopped at a party supply store to buy doom-and-gloom black decorations, appropriate for someone hitting this milestone birthday. I swung by our local bakery to pick up a cake I had ordered. Our friendly baker Bonnie chided me about the cake, which read OVER THE HILL in black frosting.

With the cake in one hand and a handful of decorations in the other, I walked through the doors of our home in an upbeat mood. When I entered the kitchen, I could not believe the mess: dishes stacked up in the sink, food all over the center island. I turned to the living room and saw MK's toys all over the floor and a heap of laundry on the sofa. It was only ninety minutes before the guests arrived. Carolyn came downstairs looking a little out of it. Maybe she'd just had a nap?

I decided to be a smart ass.

"Carolyn, I was so busy at work today that I missed the news about the tornado ripping though Sylvania. Are the kids and the rest of the family okay? Were you able to get everyone in the basement before it blew through the family room and the kitchen?"

Carolyn did not look amused in the least bit. "I didn't have time today to pick anything up," she snapped.

"Did you forget that we are having thirty people over in a couple hours?"

"I've been pretty sick today and haven't had the energy to pick up. If you're so worried about the way things look around here, you should have gotten home earlier."

"Forget it. I will do it all now. You should have called me to give me a heads-up that our home was declared a natural disaster area. I would have come home earlier."

I dove into cleaning and getting the house in good order and then moved on to decorating. Moments before the first guests were scheduled to arrive, I was on a kitchen chair trying to hook a big HAPPY BIRTHDAY onto the ceiling.

"Sean, you're not doing that right."

"Leave me alone. I'm doing my best."

"You are going to destroy the paint if you use duct tape to stick that sign up there."

"I've worked hard trying to give you a good birthday, and I don't remember asking for your opinion on how I should decorate."

"Fine."

"Fine."

We began the evening not speaking to each other.

Luckily, the dinner with her girlfriends changed her mood. While the women were at the restaurant, I wrapped the porch and the front door in black ribbon thick enough to make it difficult for them to get through. I enjoyed watching Carolyn's friends, many of whom had had several drinks, try to break through the barrier. They were laughing and seemed to enjoy the challenge.

Carolyn sat in the living room, overcome by all the presents: gift certificates for a bookstore, beautiful jewelry, and clothes. As she opened her gifts, her girlfriends discussed how turning forty made them question whether they had accomplished everything they thought they should by that age.

"I only have a few years left to be discovered," said Carolyn's friend Melanie, who wasn't forty yet. "The first time a Hollywood movie producer sees me, he will know instantly that my wit and smashing good looks are wasted as a labor and delivery nurse."

"Melanie, I think you still have a chance at fame," Carolyn said.

"Please!" said Melanie. "At this age, I'm more likely to get famous for something that would put me in the pages of some low-rent tabloid."

They all laughed, but I caught Carolyn's eye. Melanie was making us cringe. They might be seeing us in one of those later this year.

After our last guest had left, we breathed a sigh of relief. Carolyn embraced me and said, "We still have our secret."

CHAPTER 8

Maybe, Maybe Not

March 24, 2009

At this time my clients are able to provide your clients with the following information.

- *They are approximating that they live no more than 100 miles from your clients.*
- *They do have living children that are in perfect health and have experienced normal development from birth.*

Attached, please find an ultrasound picture taken on Monday, March 23, 2009. The baby was measuring 9 weeks 1 day at the time of the ultrasound, which is indicative of healthy fetal development. The heartbeat at the time of the ultrasound was 180 beats per minute, which is very healthy as well. It should also be noted that the ultrasound picture shows the disappearance of the subchorionic hematoma that was visible in prior ultrasound pictures. This is also promising progress.

Their next prenatal appointment is scheduled for Tuesday, March 31, 2009. It is scheduled for late in the afternoon, so communication regarding the results of that appointment will not occur until Wednesday, April 1, 2009.

CAROLYN

ONCE THE PREGNANCY REACHED ten weeks, I felt more confident that this baby would live, and I started to worry all the time about our embryos. I had an unsettling feeling that they were already lost. If they weren't gone, I imagined they had been damaged in the mistake.

I didn't know whether any of what I imagined was true, but the vision I had seemed so plausible. I pictured the embryologist discovering his error and rushing to the cryopreservation tanks to find out if what he feared was true. I imagined him unscrewing the tank, like one would unscrew the top of a thermos. As liquid nitrogen wafted up, he would have searched frantically for my embryos.

When he found them, I pictured him removing the catheters where my embryos were stored, a procedure that is supposed to happen just before they are thawed. He would have lifted them out of the tank and stared at them for a while. I feared that he had thrown all protocol out the window at that point, laying the catheters on the counter while he double-checked my chart, hoping and praying he was reading it wrong. My embryos would have been thawing with every second that passed. I imagined that it took him a few minutes to gather himself and put my embryos back into the tank. By then, the damage would have been done.

I would force myself to turn away from the horror of that image and hope and pray that my embryos harbored one or two more children for our family. Not all of them were likely to be viable; nevertheless, I thought, *Surely God will reward us for saving this baby. Surely there is a baby for us at the end of this nightmare.* So I prayed for them. Just like I prayed for Drew, Ryan, Mary Kate, and the baby I was carrying. I prayed that God would protect my future children and deliver them safely to me . . . sooner rather than later.

I also wanted to do something for us. For me. It felt like everything we had done since February 16 had gone toward helping this unborn child and the other family. I just wanted to have something to hope for, something to look forward to.

Long before we ever did IVF, Sean and I traveled to see a doctor in the Indianapolis area for a consultation. He had an excellent reputation and had helped friends of ours finally achieve their family after ten years of failures. He was the first doctor to recommend that we seriously consider IVF. Although we did our first IVF with our local doctor, the doctor in Indianapolis was the first one who popped into my mind as I tried to figure out what to do with our remaining embryos.

I called his practice and asked to speak to the head embryologist, who seemed very sympathetic to our situation. The plan we made was for me to pick up my embryos at the old clinic, which would place them in a portable cryopreservation tank about the size of a fire extinguisher, and then strap them into MK's car seat with bungee cords and drive them to meet with the new embryologist and doctor.

A few days after my birthday, the phone rang. I recognized the number as the Indianapolis doctor's office. I expected that it would be someone confirming all the plans for the big move. Instead, it was the embryologist. He sounded contrite as he asked me how I was doing. I sensed that something was wrong.

"After much discussion, we have decided we are unable to help you," he said.

"I'm sorry. What?"

"We are not going to be able to accept you as a patient here. So it won't be necessary for you to move your embryos here next week."

Panic washed over me.

"We don't know where else to turn," I blurted out. "We don't have a relationship with any other fertility practices. I don't even know how to start a search for a new clinic under these circumstances!" I could feel the tears streaming down my face.

"I'm sorry. I feel really bad about this. If you want, I'll look into some other options for you," the embryologist said.

"No. No. We'll figure it out. I have to go. My boys are getting off of the bus. They can't see me crying."

I shook my head as I hung up the phone, frantically brushing away tears. His office probably didn't want to be associated with us, and I couldn't blame him for that. Who would? After all, I knew I was likely to become the poster child for the humdinger of all assisted reproduction disasters.

I began wondering what I was going to do. What if no one wanted to help us? What if no one wanted to be associated with our situation? I knew we had done nothing wrong, but it was just a matter of time before the media would be all over this story. No one wanted to be mistakenly seen as the clinic that did this to us.

I could hear the boys in the kitchen rummaging around for an after-school snack. I collected myself by splashing some cool water on my face and then went downstairs with a smile on my face to help with homework and cook dinner.

To the Genetic Couple's Lawyer

April 1, 2009

Attached please find the most recent ultrasound picture provided by my clients. It was taken yesterday, March 31, 2009. As depicted in the picture, the baby is measuring 10 weeks and 3 days. The heart rate was 184 beats per minute. These are both signs of continued healthy fetal development.

My client's next prenatal appointment is scheduled for Wednesday, April 8, 2009. Results from that appointment will be forwarded that afternoon.

SEAN

SOON AFTER LEARNING that we would have to find a new clinic for our embryos, we had our weekly appointment with Kevin. Carolyn explained that she felt as though our embryos had been disregarded by everyone but us. He asked, "Are you familiar with the concept of equanimity?"

Carolyn and I shook our heads.

"Equanimity is the idea that when things are going well, we are at peace. And when things are not going well, we are at peace. The ideal in a spiritual life is to be at peace with what is and always react steadily."

We must have looked dumbfounded.

"Have you heard the story 'Maybe, Maybe Not'?"

Again, we answered no. So he told it to us.

There was a farmer who used a great horse to help him on his farm. One day his horse ran away. His neighbors said to him, "Farmer, that is awful. You lost your horse." He replied, "Maybe, maybe not."

Within a few days the farmer was surprised to find that the horse had returned—with three additional wild horses. The new horses could be quite useful on his farm. His neighbors marveled at his good fortune. "Farmer, you are so lucky. You now own several horses. You will work so much faster in your fields." The farmer replied, "Maybe, maybe not."

The next day the farmer's son tried to ride one of the wild horses but was bucked, resulting in a broken leg. The neighbors came to visit the farmer and said, "Farmer, this is tragic. Your son cannot walk." The farmer replied, "Maybe, maybe not."

Soon an army troop stormed the town, kidnapping all of the town's young men to press into service in their war. The troop was attacked, and all of the town's young men perished. The neighbors came to the farmer and said, "Farmer, you are so lucky. All of our sons have died, yet you still have yours because he was too injured to go with the soldiers." The farmer replied, "Maybe, maybe not."

This was an "aha" moment for both of us. I had never viewed the events of my life in this manner. Carolyn's eyes were lighting up as she processed the concept and the story. Was this the worst thing that had ever happened to us? I certainly thought so. Could we learn something from it? Hard to imagine, but . . . maybe, maybe not.

CAROLYN

WHEN KEVIN ASKED US if we understood the story, I said we did. To me it meant that the twists and turns of life harbor tragedies that turn into blessings and blessings that give way to tragedy. The farmer quietly accepted the twists and turns of life and waited. He didn't get too excited about anything because he knew that the world could change for him in the blink of an eye. Instead, he stayed even-keeled, accepting what life brought next and dealing with it in peace. Kevin knew that peace was what we were craving when he shared that story.

We got more than peace, however, from that story. The farmer accepted that his first impression of something as good or bad was not always a reflection of how it would affect his life, but he wasn't passive about it. He tried to make the most of what life dealt him, never being too attached to the idea of reversal or triumph.

I had been so upset that I was turning forty and this was our last chance at a baby. After that session with Kevin, I understood that this was not our last chance. I thought back to a night a few days after MK was born. I was pumping a bottle of breast milk because MK was too weak to nurse and I needed to start my supply. Suddenly I was overcome by the realization that our baby was here. My stomach was all torn up from the C-section, and I couldn't have looked or felt more terrible, but at the same time I knew we were living a dream come true. *Thank you, God. Thank you, God*, I said over and over again. We had our beautiful baby, against all the odds. Defying the dour scolding of that doctor in Cleveland, we held a miracle in our hands. Somehow I knew in my bones that my embryos had among them at least one more child. If we were going to continue to live our values, we had to find a way to give our embryos a chance at life. We needed to start the process of finding a surrogate to carry our child.

I had spoken with Sean years before about surrogacy, but he immediately rejected the idea. We were much younger then, with many years ahead of us in the world of fertility and infertility. He felt that the costs were prohibitive, and no doctor had brought up the idea or recommended that we needed surrogacy to achieve a successful pregnancy and delivery. But now all of those considerations were tossed up in the air.

The choice to start looking for a surrogate changed my feelings about the other family. I was angry at them for assuming I could immediately flip my intentions and become a surrogate. I did not want this responsibility. I resented their lack of gratitude and understanding. But here we were at the end of the first trimester, and the doctor said that there was a more than 90 percent chance that this was a viable pregnancy. I had allowed this baby to grow, and I was hopeful that we would find a young, healthy woman with a big heart who could do the same for us.

I knew Sean would not like the idea. All throughout our marriage I've known that there is a specific way to introduce new ideas: with patience. When we had Ryan, I knew early on that we would need a bigger house and a larger place for the boys to play. I had to start talking about it eighteen months before I wanted the new house to be a reality because Sean needed six or seven months to consider the idea before he warmed to it. With the surrogacy, we didn't have time to play that game. We needed to get going on this right away. I'd have to do some thinking about how to raise the subject, but we were going to have to have that conversation very soon. I knew it wouldn't go well at first. But I knew, in the end, he would agree.

As I drifted off to sleep every night I whispered to the little life growing inside of me, as I had with all of my babies, "Mama loves you, sweetie," repeating those words as I gently rubbed my belly. This baby needed to know that he or she was loved. I pictured some other woman eventually doing the same as my baby grew daily under her care. Mine was a mommy's love, a universal feeling that linked me to Shannon. I returned to feeling how worried Shannon must be for her baby, just as I would be when our surrogate was pregnant with our child. I was treating this child the way I wanted our child to be treated, and I would work harder in the future to think of Shannon in the way I would like to be honored. *Let the anger go*, I thought, rubbing with that gentle soothing touch of mothers everywhere. *Let the anger go and replace it with mother love.*

The Second Trimester

CHAPTER 9

Charting a Course

April 8, 2009 (sent)

Attached please find the most recent ultrasound picture provided by my clients. It was taken this morning and showed the baby measuring 11 weeks, 2 days. The baby's heartbeat was 180 beats per minute. These are both signs of continued healthy fetal development.

The next prenatal appointment is scheduled for Tuesday, April 14, 2009. Information from the appointment will be forwarded that afternoon.

CAROLYN

I CROUCHED DOWN next to our bed and pulled up the dust ruffle, angling my head to peer into the dim space underneath. Just at arm's reach, behind the stray socks and dust bunnies, I spotted it: a brown toiletry bag that contained the fetal heart rate monitor I bought when I was pregnant with MK. I had been blindsided by all four of my miscarriages, finding out that the baby had died only when a heartbeat couldn't be detected. I never wanted that surprise again. With the monitor, I had reassurance whenever I needed it.

A fetal heart beats fast. The wand's search through layers of fluid and tissue distorts the sound and creates a slight echo. Early on it's a flutter. As the baby grows, the beat gets stronger, quicker, and much easier to find. When I was carrying MK, I comforted myself with that sound, which mimics the galloping of a horse. In the morning and at night before bed, I'd listen to my baby galloping toward life with every beat of her heart. Where was this Little One on that journey?

Kneeling by the bed, I unzipped the pouch and found everything in its place: the monitor with its wand that looked like a small microphone, a bottle of ultrasound gel, and the stopwatch. *Maybe I shouldn't do this*, I thought. Linda had said that it was way too early for me to find the heartbeat with this equipment. If it picked up just my own heart rate and blood flow, I'd end up scaring myself. *But what if I can find it? Then I'll know the baby is growing. I'll know the baby is safe.*

I lay down on the floor next to the bed and adjusted my clothes. As I squirted the gel, gooey and cool, across my abdomen, I could hear the sounds of spring through the open windows that face the front of our property. One reason we'd bought this house was the peace it offers. The surrounding land is full of wildlife, and out here the stars in the evening skies are undimmed by city lights. As I lay on the floor searching for Little One, I heard the birds singing in the trees. We were having a warm spring. Yet until today I'd barely noticed the change in the season. I had spent much of the last two months in this room moving between the bathroom and the bed.

In the early weeks of life, the baby nestles deeply in the protection of the pelvis, and since the wand cannot pick up sound through bone, I'd have to be crafty to hear this Little One. I started scanning my lower abdomen, hearing nothing but a swooshing sound. I sucked in my breath, collapsing my abdominal cavity, and pushed hard on the wand. Still nothing.

Maybe I wasn't using enough gel. I squirted more on, making quite a mess, but I didn't care. I kept sweeping, lower and lower, until the wand was practically on the top of my pelvis. Then I pressed down and pointed it toward my toes.

Goodness, don't press too hard!

Still nothing. I started to move the wand back and forth.

Come on, Little One. Where are you hiding? Suddenly, I wanted to find this baby so badly.

I squirted on more gel, hoping it would enhance the sound. I heard a sound like wind blowing though the trees: the sound of blood flowing through my placenta. After a few minutes I pointed my toes, exhaled heavily, collapsing my lungs as far as I could to make more space to probe. And I heard it . . . faint but strong.

There you are!

I smiled broadly as I fumbled for the stopwatch. I took a fifteen-second heart rate. Forty-one times four is 164. One hundred sixty-four beats per minute.

That's pretty darn good, Little One. You must be a strong little person. You cut in line to get here. You found the heart of a family that would let you grow, and you hung on through a blood clot in your new home. Not bad for someone the size of a marble. I love you, Little One. I love you.

I lay still for a moment on the floor, savoring the discovery, content that I could have this private moment as often as I liked.

Then I thought, *I'm torturing myself, aren't I?*

Every time I sought out that sound, I grew closer to something that I'd lose. I so wanted a taste of something that was going right, to know that the baby was growing, that this child was safe.

I wiped off my stomach and the heart rate monitor, impressed by the amount of gel I'd slopped around in my search. I placed the pieces back in the toiletry bag and shoved it safely under the bed. As I stood, the spell of that time I'd shared with Little One was broken. I glanced at the clock and then to the mess of clothes heaped on the bed. After Mary Kate woke from her nap, we'd be heading out to meet Sean for an appointment with Kevin Anderson.

I had spent a ridiculous amount of time that morning trying to figure out what to wear. I was starting to show very early. I guess that's what happens when a forty-year-old mom has been pregnant three times in two and a half years. With the warmer weather, I realized that it was time to pack away the sweaters and long coats I'd used to camouflage my expansion. From the back of the closet, I had unearthed the maternity shorts I bought when I was pregnant with MK, but I couldn't find a top that fit but still disguised my shape. Before he'd left for work that morning, I asked Sean's opinion.

"Sean, what about this?" I said, showing him my profile in a T-shirt.

"Too tight."

He was right. The top part of the T-shirt fit great, but it was so tight around my abdomen that it emphasized my pregnancy. Next I tried a baby doll top, gathered at the yoke and loose around the hem.

"What about this?" I asked, twirling around in the baby doll top.

"Looks like my grandma's."

"What about this?" I'd donned a sweater that hung loose over my belly, one that had been my go-to cover-up for most of the month of March.

"Are you kidding? You'll sweat to death! You know, you might just have to hold MK if you see anyone."

So I chose the baby doll top. In truth, I just wanted to stay home. I was tired of hiding this pregnancy. I wanted to tell everyone I met that I was pregnant, but that wasn't in the cards. Also, I was ambivalent about the session. We were going to discuss our upcoming meeting with Paul and Shannon. I didn't really want to talk about it. But of course, I knew that it's those times when you don't want to see your counselor that are actually the times when you really need his help.

I glanced at my profile in the mirror. No one could see my belly in this outfit. Just in case, there would be no errands, no quick stop at the café downtown. If I went directly home after the appointment, no one would ask any questions. I scooped up MK, and we made our way to Kevin's office, where we found Sean already standing outside the door with a worried frown on his face.

SEAN

THERE WAS SO MUCH on my mind that I had starting getting stress headaches that arrived as a band of pain across my forehead. Staying organized was some help, but as I went through my day at work and to and from home or practice, all the free space in my mind churned through all we had to manage. In February I had started dictating into a recorder as I drove. My friend Marty suggested in our initial conversation that I do this to keep track of events and feelings as they occurred. Now I was so glad that I'd taken his advice. Sometimes, rather than making plans and lists, I'd just talk about what was happening and the issues we couldn't resolve. By the time we got to April I was more comfortable exploring all of the issues out loud. I came to think of this practice of recording my thoughts as a driving meditation, like my running was at night.

I had started to worry about our legal situation with the clinic. In April we were contacted by an attorney who let us know that he would be representing the clinic in the matter of the medical error. I did some research on him and discovered that he was a very well credentialed attorney. He specialized in medical malpractice defense and had an excellent record. When he and I spoke, I informed him that we had not acquired legal representation regarding the mistake. I asked him for a copy of the clinic's safety protocol and requested that he help us get Carolyn's medical records so that we could transfer our embryos and records to a new clinic. After making these requests, I patiently waited. As I drove I realized that it had been nearly eight days since I'd spoken with the attorney and he hadn't yet responded to my requests. Perhaps we needed to seek legal representation to deal with the clinic's attorney. We hoped not to have to involve attorneys in this regard, but the nonresponse indicated that we would need some help.

These legal maneuverings caused Carolyn and me to start wondering whether the clinic could be absolutely certain that a mix-up had occurred. Why were they not getting us the medical records? We had not yet been provided with evidence that our embryos were safe and secure or been given an explanation of how the mistake occurred and how it was discovered. We pictured the frantic actions that probably occurred in the lab when the doctors realized what they had done. They probably checked labels and records while adrenaline was running at full tilt. What if they had made a mistake about the mistake? One night, when we were going to sleep, this was our topic.

"They say they know where our embryos are, but how do we have proof?"

"How do they know whose baby I am carrying?" Carolyn asked. "We're planning to hand over this child to another family, but could there be an even bigger error involved? After all, if this clinic is capable of screwing it up this much, how can we be certain that there isn't an even bigger mistake? I am not turning this child over until I know it is not our genetic baby.

"It can take weeks to get a genetic match once the baby is born," Carolyn said. "This child would be in limbo until the test results come. Unless we do an amniocentesis."

"We've always said no to that," I said. "I don't want them sticking a needle in you and taking out the amniotic fluid. Even if the risks are small, they're too great."

"The odds are against me having any trouble with the test."

"We had a one-in-three-million event occur, and so I will never be convinced the odds are too low."

As I drove to work, I was beginning to see her point. If we tested the baby after birth, the baby would be in limbo for weeks without any recognized parents. I could not stand in the way of the amnio, but the concept of the test was frightening.

If the baby was confirmed to be the genetic child of the other family, we could confidently move forward and make arrangements that would ease the change of custody. I wondered how that would work. I guessed that, when we headed to the hospital for the birth, we'd have to call the lawyer as well as the doctor. By being proactive, we could ensure that our names never appeared on the birth certificate. I realized that Paul's and Shannon's names should be on the birth certificate as parents (if they were his parents!). It would be good for the child over the long term not to have a birth certificate that was a constant reminder of the mix-up.

While we had to put in place the legal planning for the change of custody, we also had to begin planning for the future of our family. That future would not involve Carolyn carrying any more children. I never in my wildest thoughts imagined having to use someone else to carry our child, but two different doctors told us that this would be Carolyn's last pregnancy. So, if we wanted to have another child within two or three years of Mary Kate, we had to choose a surrogate soon. The idea was mind-blowing. We started our family when we were just out of college, and at the rate we were going we would be attending high school graduations with the aid of walkers and canes. If much more time passed, I could definitely see Drew or Ryan pushing me there in a wheelchair. The economics were daunting, but I couldn't let money get in the way. Carolyn and I had always saved and saved for a rainy day, and now it was pouring.

I wasn't in the mood for a philosophical or religious discussion that afternoon, but I kept our commitment to see Kevin. The topic of the session that week didn't even touch on our potential future children: we were to discuss meeting the other family.

I respected Kevin and valued everything we'd learned from him in our sessions, but sometimes he made me feel inadequate when it came to the great philosophical and spiritual ideas. He usually framed an issue by starting off with a story or a saying by a great thinker or spiritual leader that we were supposed to ponder and take guidance from. Each time he would ask, "Have you heard of . . . ?" I would immediately look down and shake my head no. All of a sudden I was back in front of my eighth-grade teacher, Sister Brenda Rose, confessing that I did not study for the test.

Once in a while I was so glad when he brought up a philosopher he had referenced at a previous session. I could respond, "Of course, Kevin, who doesn't know who that is?" I was hoping just once he'd start off with something like, "Do you know anything about the Boston Celtics organization under Red Auerbach?" And I would jump off the couch and say, "Hell, yes! I read Auerbach's biography, and let me tell you a few things about his philosophy!" Not likely, but still, I could hope.

I got to Kevin's office early and was waiting outside when Carolyn arrived with MK. All of Carolyn's rest and good nutrition were paying off, and we were very hopeful that this pregnancy would go full term. The baby was growing beautifully. The images from our last ultrasound were vivid. The more detailed they were, the more we bonded with the baby. And now we were going to have to meet the parents. I had a difficult time even forming that sentence.

Kevin opened the door to his office and ushered us in. Each time we saw Kevin I was struck by the gentleness of his manner. We could come in with a significant amount of anxiety, and he seemed to be able to soothe it almost immediately. Sometimes I didn't get what he was talking about right away, but by the end of the hour it usually resonated within me.

We all took our assigned seats—Carolyn and I on the plush sofa next to one another and Kevin in a chair about five feet from us. Behind Kevin was a sliding-glass door that overlooked the courtyard of the church building. Carolyn was busy getting MK situated on the floor with some toys, so I started.

"I know we have to meet the other family eventually, but I actually don't see why it has to be now," I said. It felt right to launch immediately into what was on our minds.

"Is there something that worries you about this meeting?" he asked. "What frightens you?"

"I don't trust people I don't know, and I tread lightly when I'm not sure what's up ahead," I said. "Nothing about the situation we're in is predictable at this stage. Carolyn and I were left to read the tea leaves for a number of days after the other family knew what had happened. They didn't communicate with us, and I was unsure of the reason for the delay. And when the letter came, they said they were grateful, but it also focused on themselves and their struggles. This makes me even more cautious. If Shannon was carrying our baby, I would have offered anything I could to help. I don't want to make judgments, just observations."

As Kevin contemplated what I had said the silence became uncomfortable. I stared at the fountain and focused on the trickling water.

Then Carolyn spoke up with her usual unsparing honesty.

"I make judgments," she said. "I harbor such resentment. I feel like I am being used by them. They've done nothing, and they get everything? I'm jealous."

It pained me to hear her say such harsh things, because she has such a huge heart. But in my book, it's not so much what we say but what we do that counts. Carolyn's actions were all about compassion and caring for this other family.

Carolyn started to cry. I put my arm around her. I didn't know what to say then. Carolyn's tears sometimes have a way of doing that to me. I feel helpless and like there's nothing I can do to help make her hurt go away. And there's nothing I want more in that moment than to make it go away.

"You know why I really don't want to meet them? Because I know me," Carolyn continued through her sobs. "When Paul and Shannon become real people to me, I will want to help them and want to like them. Our disaster was their miracle, and after we meet, I will want to find a way to be happy for them. I'm not ready to be happy for them. I'm not even ready to like them. Part of me hopes they are awful. That way, I'd be justified in all the terrible things I've been thinking about them."

"You see that picture hanging on the wall behind me?" Kevin indicated the M. C. Escher print called *Sky and Water*, a black-and-white drawing of doves ascending; gradually, as the eye travels downward, the shapes morph into fish descending. The fish point downwards, as if the only direction left to swim is into darkness.

"I use that picture with clients who need to understand the depths of grief and despair. The fish in the bottom left-hand corner exists at depths of suffering that most people never experience. One cannot feel more darkness than where that fish is. That is where I think you are. You are being swallowed by grief and sadness. In the range of difficult human experiences, what you are going through is comparable to a death."

Up to that point, I couldn't have described the experience. Kevin really got it. Death. There would be no showing, burial, or funeral where a broad group of people would come together to grieve a life. It would be a death only to us and no one else. A very lonely loss. Life would go on for this child, but just not in our world.

"You are that fish, and the objective is to get the two of you to start to swim upwards. You need to move from that deep dark corner, toward the light. Unfortunately, the ascent from that depth of despair is going to take a long, long time. This will not be over for you in the near future. It will be hard work, but you can ascend. You can with time and by staying with the work of healing."

Carolyn had mentioned that print after one of our previous sessions with Kevin, but I'd never taken such a long look at it. Kevin did not have any quick answers. But he did ask good questions.

"Did you know that there are two interpretations of the Passion of Christ?" Kevin asked. I immediately thought, *I should have joined that damn Bible study class when it was offered.* I looked at Kevin and sheepishly shook my head no again.

"The dominant view is that God sent Jesus down to suffer and die for the people," Kevin said. "The other view is that Jesus lived His life and developed a huge following and, through a series of choices, eventually saw that those choices would lead to great suffering for Him and to death. He decided to not turn away from it, even though it meant the cross."

I was captivated.

"The first view is difficult to understand, when you really think about it, because what father sends his only son to suffer and die?" Kevin continued. "The second view is a more humane view of Christ, yet it does not take away from the passion. In fact, it elevates it further, because He could have stopped or changed His course, but He did not. He accepted the suffering and made the sacrifice. I cannot pretend to know what you are going through, but you made a choice that meant suffering and sacrifice. I want you to look at the pain you are feeling in that context. You are experiencing some of life's most profound suffering."

As was usual after our sessions with Kevin, we did not leave with definitive answers. Would we meet the other family? Carolyn and I now had a platform from which to launch further discussions. We were not yet ready to answer that question, but we would be soon. I escorted Carolyn to her car and stood with her as she placed MK in her car seat. As she did these simple tasks, the basic work of modern motherhood, I watched her pull herself together for the drive. It was remarkable to see her fully experience her sorrow and anxiety about meeting the other family and then reclaim her equanimity before putting the key in the ignition. Maybe I wouldn't have stopped to appreciate this simple action if it hadn't been for Kevin's advice to acknowledge the grace in what we were doing.

I got into my car and took a deep breath. I wanted to see and feel the grace, but all I felt was pressure and stress. There were so many appointments related to this crisis; it was practically a full-time job, on top of the one I already had. The newest area that involved more meetings was the search for legal representation on the medical mistake.

We had recently done a significant amount of research to select an attorney to represent us. We had narrowed the search down to a very reputable attorney, Brian McKeen. When Brian sat down with Carolyn and me for a meeting in Toledo in April, three things captured me beyond his impressive credentials. Before he asked any legal questions or provided us with any opinion, he said, "I am impressed with what you are doing for this baby and the other couple. If you don't hire me, I will still feel very fortunate that I had the opportunity to meet you." This statement spoke to his priorities and his character. Second, Brian had a passion for his work and asked excellent questions and listened intently. Third, Brian had an immense knowledge and understanding of this area of law, the medical terminology, and everything about pregnancy.

Within forty-eight hours of the meeting, we hired Brian as our lead attorney; Marty Holmes Jr. would be involved in a supportive role. Their task was to work with the clinic to come to a reasonable settlement regarding the mistake and to try to achieve that without filing a lawsuit. Carolyn and I felt very fortunate to have such able representation.

A few days later we continued the conversation about meeting the genetic parents, this time with both Marty Holmes Sr. and Jr. and with our family law attorney, Mary Smith, at the Holmes law offices in downtown Toledo. When we arrived, the receptionist escorted us to a huge conference room with a table large enough to seat sixteen people.

Sitting there before the lawyers arrived felt odd, as if we were little kids in Dad's big office. I guess that thought came to me because I'd known Marty since we were kids, and I'd known his dad Marty Sr. just as long, at a time in my life when I thought of him as a towering figure. Marty Jr. was part of my close-knit high school group that had been so loyal to each other through the years. I knew from experience that Marty would have my back. Marty had been there for me consistently since I called him on February 17, providing not only legal support but, more importantly, life support. There were few people in the world I trusted as much as the Holmes family. They were the perfect people to advise us about my big fear that the media would invade our lives and badger us endlessly.

When this issue came up after they arrived for the meeting, they told us that the fact that our house was in a private subdivision would be a big help in maintaining our privacy. Marty Sr. warned us that the press could be aggressive in pursuing us at home and at work and that we needed to prepare ourselves for this possibility.

"You'd be surprised what some of them are willing to do," Marty Sr. said.

Carolyn didn't find this reassuring. She hated even thinking about it. I looked over at her and saw that she was playing with her bracelet. Her eyes were far away as she took the clasp that held her bracelet apart and then fitted it back together again and again.

"You have to be pristine in the comments that you make to the press," Marty Holmes Sr. said. "Speak slowly, clearly, and concisely."

After hearing Mr. Holmes's advice, I had a feeling that we might need to hire someone else to help us handle the media part of this soon. Another task to add to the binder.

We shifted topics to the upcoming meeting with the genetic family.

"I think we should start from the best possible outcome and work our way toward that as a goal," said Marty Jr. "The best-case scenario is the two families completely at peace with what has transpired. A great visual is the two families standing arm in arm after the birth in front of the hospital for a happy photo as they thank you for all that you've done."

"You've got to be joking," Carolyn said. I could see her eyes starting to fill with tears. "I can't even imagine getting through the delivery, let alone standing in front of the hospital arm in arm. That idea is incomprehensible to me."

"That might be the ideal," I said, backing Carolyn up, "but I cannot imagine the shape we will be in at that time."

"I think a home run for the other family is for you to find a way to let the baby go with no strings attached," Marty Jr. added.

"What is our home run?"

"We don't have one," Carolyn stated.

"Carolyn, do you know how grateful this other mother is going to be to you?" Mary asked. "Maybe they'll even make you god-parents."

"Maybe," Carolyn said. "Maybe not."

"Their attorney has assured me that they are really nice people," Mary said, adding, "They are desperate. Every time I send a communication their lawyer tries to confirm that they are going to get their baby. I think they are really suffering."

"We are not people who go back on our word," I asserted. "When we say we will hand the child over to them at delivery, that is exactly what we are going to do." As I made this strong statement, it occurred to me that this was one place that had no "maybe, maybe not."

"So let's set a date to meet them," Marty Jr. said.

I looked at Carolyn. "I can see that this meeting would give them much-needed relief at some level. If meeting us helps them, then we will put our fears aside and do it."

"I agree, but I think you need to know that meeting them does not change our situation," Carolyn said.

"You don't have to tell them everything," Marty Jr. advised. "Tell them just as much as you feel comfortable sharing and not anything more than that."

On the way home Carolyn and I decided that we'd work on an outline of what we wanted to communicate to the genetic parents. To me it was important to limit what we told them to what they needed to know to reassure them that their baby was well cared for and that we would be handing the baby over in the hospital with no strings attached. (In fact, Carolyn and I wanted to attach all kinds of strings to this child so that we could ensure that we would have a long-term relationship, but we thought that would not be right.) We needed to stay away from any topic unrelated to those two issues until we became more comfortable with them.

I was sure that they expected that meeting us and finding out more about who we were would lessen their stress about the pregnancy and their child. But I knew that the meeting might just do the opposite. Learning about Carolyn's health history would not leave anyone feeling comfortable about her pregnancy. I found that I did not want Paul and Shannon to feel more anxious than they already did about the health and well-being of their child. Carolyn might think it was mean not to be completely open with them about everything, but I wanted to protect them. We'd have to find a middle ground.

Note Sent to the Genetic Parents' Lawyer by Our Lawyer on April 14, 2009

Attached please find the latest ultrasound picture from today. It pictures the baby at 12 weeks, 2 days development with a heartbeat of 167 beats per minute. The next prenatal appointment and ultrasound are scheduled for Tuesday, April 21, 2009. Results will be forwarded that afternoon.

In addition, my clients are requesting a meeting with your clients the week of April 24, 2009. If they'd like to as well, please get back to me to schedule a mutually convenient time.

CAROLYN

THE SUNDAY NIGHT BEFORE our meeting with the other family, we sat in our bedroom with the door closed, rehearsing how we would behave when we met them. Sean had taken out one of his massive binders. He has an archaic organizational system that makes me crazy. It is archaic in the sense that it exists on paper. Lots and lots of paper, slipped into acrylic sleeves and slid into a binder. I'm not exactly sure where Sean shops for his binders, because they are the biggest binders I have ever seen. I have to buy binders when I buy school supplies for the boys, so I've seen the binder section of the office supply store. Sean's binders are not from the stores I shop in. I think he special-orders them, as the size of these monsters exceeds the normal four-inch jumbos found on retail shelves.

Sean has a binder for absolutely everything in his life. He has a tax binder, a business/personal goals binder, an estate/financial-plan binder, and binders for every sport he coaches. The binders are all titled, carefully labeled, and divided into sections that make sense to him. Every Friday evening he unloads his "binder system" in our home office, stacking them on the floor and sometimes on the otto-man of the chair in the office—not my first choice of spots to store those bulky things.

The day Sean walked in with a new six-inch binder and a brand-new package of acrylic sleeves, I pretended not to notice until I saw the title of the new jumbo binder: "Sean and Carolyn's CF File." I knew immediately that this binder was for us—for this baby and this situation.

"What's that?" I asked him.

"It's a binder for this mess. We have to keep everything organized. We need to make sure every record of what we are going through is kept. You never know when we will need this stuff again."

I knew he was right. We were incurring massive expenses: med-ical visits, prescription costs, legal bills, therapist expenses, lost time at work for Sean, and God only knows what using a surrogate was going to cost us. Even though I knew the binder was a good idea, I also was acutely aware that what I was going through couldn't be charted or graphed. There were no receipts to be filed that docu-mented my grief. Sean could special-order the biggest binder in the whole world, but it would never be large enough to hold my broken heart.

Sean sat in a chair with his "CF" binder in hand as I lay on the bed. From one of the plastic sleeves he took copies of the outline we'd developed in the week since we met with the lawyers. We'd decided that Sean would go first and speak about his family history, and then I would describe mine plus our infertility struggles. We would talk about our children next, but when we thought about how that would go, questions came up.

"Are we going to tell them our kids' names?" Sean asked.

"I hadn't thought of that. I guess."

"I don't think we should. In fact, I don't think we should tell them our last name."

Thinking we'd surely introduce ourselves using our last name, I asked, "Why not? They are going to figure it out eventually. It would be rude not to tell them. They'd think we don't trust them."

"We do not know them well enough to trust or not trust them," Sean pointed out. "I want to be very cautious until we know them better, and protecting our privacy seems prudent. I think we'll be able to draw conclusions as the meeting progresses."

"Sean, that is ridiculous. We have to tell them our last names. We can keep the kids' names private."

"Okay, we will share our last names with them. Maybe I am going too far with the privacy thing," Sean conceded.

He was still trying to protect us. Sean was assuming that maybe they'd be done with us when they got what they wanted. So why should we reveal more than we had to? I thought he was being paranoid. He thought he was being realistic.

We continued on through the script, each speaking our part. When we discussed the logistics surrounding the delivery, my voice began cracking.

"I don't know how I'm going to do this. I don't think I can look at her. How am I going to do that?"

"Try not to look her in the eye. Look at something else. Like her chin."

This made me laugh. Like I was going to stare at her chin and not see her eyes that would only be a few inches away. "Maybe I'll stare at her neck. I bet she'll wear a necklace. I'll stare at that."

"Well, just don't stare at her chest. That would be rude."

I burst out laughing again. Sean's quick wit never fails me. Ever.

We went through the outline three times, adding a few things that I had forgotten. That was it. There was nothing else we could do to prepare. I went to bed grateful for Sean's meticulous preparations. I knew I would be a wreck, but having that thorough outline in my hand would ground me. I slid into bed next to Sean and faced his strong back, his broad shoulders. Together through these three months we had been to frightening places, feeling the kind of bone-shaking fear you wouldn't wish on anyone. We had cried together more in this short time than we had for the sixteen years of our marriage. And today we were laughing like goofy teenagers. *I love my husband*, I thought. *There is no one else I'd rather have at my side.*

CHAPTER 10

An Anxious Introduction

CAROLYN

"SEAN, AM I SUPPOSED to extend my hand to Shannon when she enters the room? Or do you think she'll extend hers first? Oh . . . wait. We will be in the room already . . . right. They are bringing them to us? I guess we'll just stand up and be polite, right?"

We were in the car on our way to meet the genetic family.

"Marty and Mary will lead them in. We will stand and shake their hands."

"We decided to tell them our last names. Didn't we?"

"Carolyn. We covered all of this. And if it doesn't work out the way we planned, I think we'll improvise just fine. It's not rocket science."

Sean was right. I could manage a simple introduction, but then again, there was nothing simple about meeting Shannon and Paul. I still didn't want to look her in the eye, and I knew my smile would not be genuine. In fact, I don't think I had ever dreaded an event more in my life. My hands were wringing wet from my mounting anxiety. I wiped my palms on my skirt and straightened my blouse. I had spent a lot of time trying to decide what to wear to this meeting. If I was too professional looking, I might seem standoffish or look like I was trying to come off as aloof. But I didn't want to look like a dumpy woman at the mall in an old sweat suit. A skirt and blouse was my middle ground.

Oddly enough, it didn't really matter what I had on, since I felt as though I was about to appear before them naked. I felt so exposed. We hadn't even told our families about this, and these strangers would get a front-row seat to our pain and to my physiology. And as irrational as it seemed, I felt like Shannon was coming to the meeting to get part of my body, an intimate part of me, and that both of them were coming to take my baby away.

I had vowed that I would never let them see my sadness, but as Sean and I drove to the Holmes law offices, I was petrified that I wouldn't be able to control my emotions. I was tired of acting like everything was normal as I went through a world that was teetering and heaving. I didn't want to hear Shannon talk, see her smile, have to endure her explaining that she knew how we felt. I didn't want to meet the mother of my baby.

Sean started to pull into the parking garage underneath the law offices.

"Hey, don't park here!"

"Why? Why wouldn't I park here?"

"Because. What if they parked next to us? I don't want to walk to our cars together after the meeting. That would be awkward. Park a few blocks away."

Sean rolled his eyes at me and turned the car back out into traffic so that he could find a parking spot a few blocks away.

When we signed in at the reception desk, I carefully studied the registration sheet.

"What are you doing?"

"I want to see their signatures."

"Okay."

"Looks like only Paul signed in. And it only says 'Paul.' I wanted to see their last name."

We got in the elevator, and I realized I was shaking. I remem-

bered Kevin telling us that animals shake uncontrollably when
threatened because the shaking allows them to release stress, and
that it usually lasts a few hours after the danger passes. I held up my
hand to watch it quiver and wondered how many hours it would
take for this to stop.

We entered the law firm through the large glass doors, and the
receptionist escorted us to a different conference room from where
we'd met a few weeks before. We took our places at a large wooden
table facing the door that Shannon and Paul would enter.

"Are you okay?" Sean asked as we sat down.

"No. But what does it matter?"

"Is there anything I can do?"

"Tie me down because I am repressing an urge to run from the
room, out of the building, and into the street. I don't think I can talk."

"Remember, you don't have to. They are going first. I asked for
that."

I looked at Sean, grateful that he had the forethought to ask for
that so I could collect myself after they entered. Marty Holmes Sr.
and Mary Smith came in to ask us if we had any last questions.

"Have you met them?" I asked Mary.

"Yes. They are very nice. I'm going to go and get them."

I nodded and sat back down, clenched Sean's hand, and prayed.

Please, God, help me. Please, God, help me.

It was a simple prayer, but it was all I could manage.

Breathe. Just breathe. Inhale, exhale. Slowly. It's going to be okay.

When the door opened, Sean and I stood as Mary entered with
Paul, Shannon, and their attorney, Ellen. I could hardly feel my
legs beneath me. I fixated on Shannon, who was dressed casually
in a black sweater with a scoop neck, not at all the woman I had
pictured. She was shorter than me, and she had a friendly and very
casual demeanor about her. As we all took our seats, I struggled to
find a place to look.

Not in her eyes, Carolyn. Not at the floor. Ah . . . a necklace.

Lo and behold, she wore a silver necklace.

Perfect. I'll stare at that.

Shannon spoke first, as planned. She talked rapidly, and her hands gestured enthusiastically as she spoke. I confess I wasn't hanging on her every word. I listened for just a few things. I wanted her to say thank you for saving our baby. *I heard her say she was grateful we'd agreed to continue the pregnancy.* I wanted her to tell me that she understood how awful our predicament was and that she appreciated the choice we made. *I heard her say that it was one thing to say you are pro-life, but another to walk your talk and the fact that we were doing so spoke to our character.* I wanted her to say that she couldn't imagine how grief-stricken we were, and if there was anything she could do to help to please let her know. *I heard her say how grief-stricken they were to learn that another woman would be pregnant with their baby.*

She believed that the mistake must have happened because her maiden name, which she hadn't legally changed at the time of the last transfer, was Savage and her embryos had been labeled "Savage-Morell."

"Do you think you and I are related?" she asked Sean, smiling brightly.

I think the last quarter-ounce of blood in Sean's face drained out then.

"No, I don't have any relatives in Michigan," Sean said adamantly, which surprised me. Sean has more than fifty cousins on the Savage side of his family.

"You never know," I suggested. "You could be distant relatives."

"Nope," he insisted vigorously. "We have no family in Michigan. None."

Shannon explained that she and Paul had tried to start a family immediately after they wed seven years ago. After two miscarriages, they tried IVF in 2006 and got their twins on the first try. One of the other embryos frozen then was the baby I was carrying.

I was overcome with sympathy for the Morells, just as I had

feared I would be. I could hear in her voice how difficult infertility was for them, as it is for everyone. Miscarriages are brutal, and they'd had two. Then I tried to communicate our experience, describing our family and our history of infertility.

"My family lived in Grosse Pointe, Michigan, until I was nine," I said.

"Oh, we lived there just after we were married," she said.

We recounted our ten-year struggle to conceive, our complicated history of premature delivery. Shannon was silent through that part of the chronology. I may have frightened her. I think I saw a flash of surprise pass through her eyes when I explained that we had three children, two of whom were nearly teenagers. She was more vocal when we detailed our excellent prenatal care and how we were taking every precaution with this pregnancy. She was an eager and active listener, chiming in when she identified something we had in common. When I named the hospital we would deliver at, Shannon interrupted.

"Do you want your kids to meet the baby?"

That simple question flooded me with emotions. Of course I wanted my kids to meet the baby, but I wanted so much more than that. I wanted my kids to know the baby. I wanted to know the baby. Suddenly I was frightened again. Was she saying that once they had the baby we'd never see them again?

They wouldn't do that to us. That would be cruel. No, they'll like us and want to keep us in their lives.

In a flash, my thoughts turned to a scene of my boys and Mary Kate gathering around my hospital bed to marvel at our special delivery. I never imagined that my children would not know this child, but I also knew that we wouldn't ask Paul and Shannon for visitation rights. We would never invite ourselves into their lives or the life of this child. The future of our relationship with my baby was in their hands, and I was not sure what she was saying. All of these thoughts flew through my mind in a matter of seconds, and before I knew it my eyes were filled with tears. Sean must have sensed my agony.

"That is so far off in the distance. We just aren't ready to think about delivery scenarios yet."

Good. Good job. I can't talk. I don't know how to answer that question without crying. Thank you, Sean. Thank you for saving me.

SEAN

PAUL SAT ACROSS THE TABLE from me and grimaced regularly. I could tell he was unbelievably uncomfortable. I wondered if he felt bad for us, or if he was so frightened of saying the wrong thing that he said nothing. Sometimes sitting quietly and listening is the right thing to do. Carolyn and I had our outlines clutched tightly in our hands.

The first moment we all bonded was in speaking about the doctor and clinic that had put all of us in this situation. I told them about the doctor's call to me and driving home to inform Carolyn and the voice-mail messages from him. Although Paul hardly said anything during the meeting, he spoke up then to express the hope that I'd documented those calls. I guess it is up for interpretation what he meant by expressing that, but I believe he hoped that I'd saved the messages the doctor left, or that I'd written down exactly what he said in our conversations, for legal purposes.

We did agree on my number one concern: privacy. I let them know that to date we had told only a few individuals who were bound by privilege, including a priest, a counselor, and attorneys. Before I could finish my thought, Shannon swiftly said, "I agree. How are we going to keep it that way?"

"I've thought about this a lot since February 16," I said, "and I know there is no way that we can keep a pregnancy private."

"We haven't told anyone but our lawyer," Shannon said.

"The day we found out about this we knew that the day would come when we would have to share with those around us what had happened," I said. "Pregnancy is a public event, and we're very involved in our church and the kids' school and the business community. We are not in a position to hide a pregnancy, nor are we comfortable with that idea."

"You could just tell everyone that Carolyn was serving as a surrogate for someone else," Shannon suggested.

I could feel Carolyn tensing up next to me. Anytime one referred to her pregnancy as a surrogacy, it enraged her.

"We are not going to lie about this. We are going to be genuine. We have decided to not terminate the pregnancy and to not fight for custody. After making those two decisions, it would not be consistent of us to start lying about everything else. We will be telling family and friends the truth in the coming weeks once Carolyn is visibly showing the pregnancy, and I am sure it will spread from there. Rest assured that we will keep your identity private forever if that is your request."

"We hardly told anyone about our IVF," Shannon said. "And one of the people I did tell was very critical about our choice to use IVF. If you are Catholic, aren't you worried what people in your church will say?"

"We think our friends and community will look at it differently," I said. "We think we're doing the right thing. The fact that the Church doesn't approve of IVF was something we considered, but in the end we decided it shouldn't prevent us from expanding our family. Plus, we can't control our church's reaction."

I am not sure they liked this approach, but I described our decision as strongly and with as much conviction as I could.

As the meeting was breaking up we promised to keep them informed about the pregnancy. They asked for contact information, but we declined to give it to them. I knew we would eventually, but I explained that we wanted to discuss how the meeting went and how we would move on from here. Shannon frantically wrote down every phone number they had, and their address, and handed the information to Carolyn. We thanked them for coming and wished them a safe drive home.

When the door shut behind them, we all let out a collective sigh of relief. "They seemed nice and normal, and the meeting went as well as could be expected, don't you think?" Mary said. We talked with the lawyers about the meeting for an hour or so before leaving for home. In the elevator, Carolyn looked exhausted.

"Well, what do you think?" I asked her.

"I think I'm glad it's over. I'm still pregnant with a baby that I'm not going to be allowed to keep. Now at least I know who is coming to take the baby away."

"Do you feel better about anything?"

"I'm proud of us. I got through it without crying. We probably made them feel better."

"It went well. I wonder what will happen next?"

"I don't know, and frankly," she held up her hand to demonstrate the quiver that was still controlling it, "I am really wondering how long it will take me to stop shaking."

As we made our way to our car Carolyn seemed to start relaxing and even showed a smile. Maybe being in the fresh air and out of that building gave her a sense of release.

"Shannon has beautiful blue eyes and a kind smile," Carolyn remarked. She too was reviewing the meeting and trying to find reassurance there. "I can tell she has a lot of energy in her. Seeing as how she is a teacher of eighth graders, she's probably a very patient person. I bet if she and I worked in the same school, we'd be friends."

If meeting the other family gave Carolyn some peace and helped Paul and Shannon, then the encounter was a success. They were now real to us, just people in an extraordinary situation, probably hoping and praying that they wouldn't say or do the wrong thing. The meeting had made them less of an unknown. As we got in my car, I was starting to think that maybe we could all work together to get to a better place.

CHAPTER 11

Sharing the Hurt, Feeling the Love

CAROLYN

THE FEELING OF RELIEF we got from our initial meeting with the Morells was short-lived, eaten up by the pressure around revealing our predicament to those we loved. The ordeal would take two days, starting with our parents, moving from there to Sean's siblings and their spouses, followed by phone calls to my brothers. The next day we planned to tell the boys, shortly before we called our friends together in a meeting room at our church. The schedule was exhausting, but once these two days came to a close, I wouldn't have to hide our secret anymore. Best of all, I could finally stop dressing like we lived at the Arctic Circle.

For Sean, the most intimidating meeting of the four was going to be the one where we told our parents, particularly my dad. Sean remembered clearly the day in the hospital corridor when my father looked him sternly in the eye and said, "No more babies." We also remembered the look on his face when he found out I was pregnant with Mary Kate. He loves MK with all his heart and is a wonderful grandpa to her. But when he found out we were taking on another pregnancy, I could see that he was surprised and not jubilant.

My dad was a university attorney and did a little bit of every kind of law. The cases that really rattled him were those in which he defended the university hospital against malpractice suits. He'd seen the catastrophic consequences of medical sloppiness and carelessness. There was no predicting how he would act when he found out about this situation. I just hoped he could contain his temper when he found out that his daughter was the victim of such a careless error. So did Sean. When he rehearsed this meeting with Marty Holmes Sr., Sean sweated through his shirt. We hoped that if we had my dad in the room with my mom and Sean's mom Kate, Dad wouldn't completely blow his stack.

We came up with a great reason to get my parents to come from Michigan to visit us. Drew was competing in an important 5K race at school that he was likely to win. We invited them to be there when he crossed the finish line. The race was a yearly tradition at the kids' school, the culmination of a week of inspirational talks about not using drugs and taking a "Positive Direction" in everything in life. Drew had been training hard and was running well. Sean thought he might even break the unofficial race record, and my parents were glad to be asked to witness this event. I asked them to arrive at 1:00 P.M. the day before to baby-sit MK so I could attend "a parent event" at Drew's school. I lured Kate to the house at the same time under the same pretext. I felt bad lying to them, but there was no easy way to get them together at that time.

That afternoon my mom and dad arrived right on schedule. We chatted for a few minutes, then broke off when Sean came in.

"Taking long leisurely lunches these days, Sean? Uh . . . I thought you would be back at the office guarding my money!" My dad joked with Sean because he knew Sean never took lunches.

"Well, Byron, that is the beauty of having 'people,'" Sean said with a wry smile. "I guard your money most of the day, but when I'm gone, I assign my employees to guard it in two-hour shifts. We are on watch twenty-four hours a day."

We were all laughing when the door opened again, and Kate walked in.

"Byron? Linda? What a surprise. What are you all doing here?"

And there we stood. Our parents looked confused as to why all of them were there, while I looked like the cat that ate the canary.

"Well, we have something to tell you. There is no event at Drew's school today," I said. "We just wanted to talk to you together, and we couldn't think of another way to get you here without tricking you. So, sorry. Please, sit down."

I could see how frightening this sounded. The proof was all over my mother's wide-eyed face. Obediently they walked into the family room. My mom sat on the couch next to me. Dad pulled a wooden rocking chair from the corner, and Kate sat in a chair. Sean sat down next to her.

"No one is sick, we're not getting a divorce, and no one is going to jail," Sean started off.

"Well, that's good, I guess," my dad said, still looking scared.

"Look, this is not easy to say, so I'm going to say it. You all know that MK was conceived through IVF?" Sean said.

They nodded.

"Well, we had leftover embryos from that IVF that were frozen. This past February, Carolyn and I did a frozen embryo transfer, and she is now sixteen weeks pregnant."

My mom squealed with joy.

"Hold on, Linda. This is not good news. Apparently, when they thawed the embryos, they pulled the wrong ones. They transferred another couple's embryos into Carolyn. She is pregnant with another couple's baby."

I had been staring at the floor the entire time, feeling my cheeks burn with nervousness. When Sean finished, I looked up at my dad, whose jaw was hanging wide open. His face was beet red, as if he was struggling to contain his temper. Kate had her hand over her mouth in shock.

"Oh, Carolyn!" my mom said softly, her voice cracking as her eyes filled with tears. She shook her head back and forth, refusing to accept this was so. "Is this true?"

I shook my head up and down indicating yes.

"And the other couple wants this baby," I continued, trying to erase any erroneous thought they might be having that we were going to get a baby out of this. "They are going to take this baby upon delivery, and we have agreed to allow that to happen without a fight."

Sean described how we found out about the error, told them the doctor had asked us to abort but we refused, and added that we had met Paul and Shannon and they were nice and truly wanted this baby.

"Where are your embryos?" my dad blurted out.

"We have been told they are still in cryopreservation. We are working on moving them to a different facility," I said.

"Your health comes first, Carolyn. You know that, right? Your health comes before this baby's." My dad wanted reassurance that I wasn't going to martyr myself. "You have three other children to raise, and you are very important to those children."

"Of course, Dad. Just like my other pregnancies. My health comes first."

Sean continued to explain everything that we had done to protect ourselves, how we were proceeding legally with reputable attorneys in Brian McKeen and Marty, and how we had chosen to keep this a secret for as long as we could.

"You were pregnant in Florida?" my mom asked, incredulous. "I can't believe you didn't tell us. I can't believe you went all this time keeping this to yourselves. I'm so sorry you were alone in this."

"You don't know how many times I wanted to call you," I said. "But we had to keep this a secret in case I miscarried. We didn't want you to be upset unnecessarily if I lost this baby."

An hour later we were still answering questions, particularly my father's questions, about malpractice and the legal process, when MK woke from her nap. I brought her down to play on the family room floor while we continued our conversation. While I was sitting next to MK, I looked up at my dad and saw that he was thumbing through

Brown Bear, Brown Bear, a children's board book, as he listened. He turned page after page, pretending to look intently at the illustrations. I realized he was in shock. He held that book the entire time. He was sad. We were all sad. We were a pitiful bunch that afternoon.

We wrapped up the meeting before the boys got home from school, as we thought they'd find it weird that all of their grandparents had been summoned to their home for . . . what? an afternoon cup of coffee? Before Kate left, we asked her if it would be okay to call an emergency meeting of all of Sean's siblings and their spouses at her home that evening. We didn't want to meet at our house because we weren't going to tell the boys until the next day after school. Kate agreed, and Sean immediately made eight phone calls requesting that his siblings and their spouses be at their mom's at eight o'clock that night. Sean thought if he gave his siblings only a few hours' notice, we would limit their worry time. He told each of them what he had told our parents: that we weren't sick, getting divorced, or going to jail.

Although we'd just dropped a considerable bombshell in our living room, we had to resume our "everything's just fine" posture for a carbo-loading dinner with Drew that his school was hosting. It was the special "night before the run" meal, and the school always invited an outstanding inspirational speaker to address the crowd before dinner. The original speaker had a family emergency and had to cancel, so the replacement speaker was going to be a surprise.

Drew, Sean, and I arrived at the very last minute so we could avoid any small talk before the event started. We slid into a seat in the back and heard the crowd buzzing with speculation about the speaker. When they announced that it was Mrs. Jackie Frisch, I couldn't believe my luck, as I was sure she would have a message that I needed to hear that night. Jackie is the mother of ten boys and suffers from a rare and debilitating disease that threatens her life daily. In the face of her ailment, Jackie and her husband found the strength in their hearts to adopt seven Haitian orphans—all boys—now her sons. Last year, in an episode of *Extreme Home Makeover*, the wizards from that show whipped up a beautiful new home for Jackie and her family. She is also an ordained minister, and one amazing lady.

That evening Jackie talked about gratitude and love and how grateful she was that God had chosen her to suffer from her sickness. Her illness made her love every single minute of every day she spent with her family in her home. She talked of her seven Haitian boys and three biological sons, who now filled her life with love and ate her out of house and home. Yes, her life was tough. Yes, they didn't have much money, and she worried about her health, but she exuded love. And the love made her happy.

The amazing thing about hearing Jackie talk was that it made me think that I needed to catch her fever of love. I needed help leaving my own pity party.

You need to be peaceful like her. You need to stop feeling sorry for yourself. If she can get up every day and face her fears, you surely can get through this pregnancy.

We left the carbo-loading dinner a little early, telling Drew we had to meet up with some friends. We dropped him off and headed to Kate's for our next meeting.

SEAN

Carolyn and I spoke little as we made the two-mile drive to my mom's house on a perfect spring evening. We planned to arrive at her house a few minutes after 8:00 so we wouldn't have to make small talk as we waited. I parked in front of Mom's, and Carolyn and I paused to take one last look at our reflection in the car window before we entered the house.

As I surveyed the living room, I counted my siblings and their spouses, most of whom were dressed casually in workout gear, to make sure that everyone was there. We are an athletic family, a family of runners and basketball players, but the feeling in the room wasn't our usual jocularity. We were gathered in the same room where year after year we had opened Christmas presents and hunted for Easter eggs, but the mood that night was nervous and a bit somber. When the whole family is together with the grandkids, we are forty-strong. My mom and dad have quite a legacy. They raised us kids to be fiercely independent, but as exemplified that night, if anyone needed help, we would drop everything at a moment's notice. My family knew that a meeting being called like this had to be about something serious.

Everyone had instinctively formed into a circle around the two chairs that my mom had positioned in a corner of the living room. They looked like the "hot seats." My mom told us that one of my brothers was running late. To avoid awkwardness, Carolyn and I ducked into the nursery that my mom keeps for her grandkids. I was so nervous in that nursery. I just wanted to get this over with. Soon after that, everyone was seated, and we entered. Dusk was beginning to settle outside. The room was chilly and dim, lit only by a few lamps.

Of all the family members there, the one Carolyn was most concerned about was JoAnn. My brother Kevin, her husband, was out of town, so she was taking this in alone. She was also the only person who knew Carolyn was pregnant because she was the one who had watched MK the day of our embryo transfer. Therefore, she was the person we felt the worst about, because we'd let her believe we were pregnant with our child. She and Kevin are MK's godparents. JoAnn had been ecstatic about the pregnancy and told us how she couldn't wait to get her hands on our next baby so she could cuddle and spoil him or her the way any good aunt would.

"Carolyn and I really appreciate you dropping everything to come here tonight," I said. "On February 6, Carolyn underwent a frozen embryo transfer. On February 16, the doctor called to inform me that they mistakenly transferred another couple's embryos and that Carolyn was pregnant with someone else's genetic child."

I looked up at JoAnn, who was as pale as a ghost. My sister Kelly, who is just a year older than Carolyn, held her hands over her eyes and slid a little lower in her chair with every sentence I spoke. I was glad when I was almost done because I thought she might fall on the floor. I looked at my brother Scott, who was sitting directly across the room from us gripping his forehead. My oldest brother John looked like he might get sick.

I noticed Carolyn was beginning to shake when she started her remarks. She did fine until she got to the sentence "We have been devastated by this." She got as far as "devastated" and started to cry. JoAnn practically hurdled the couch in an attempt to get her Kleenex. My mom started sobbing when she saw Carolyn begin to cry. My mom is the consummate caretaker and matriarch of the family, and I am certain she internalized our pain at that moment. The word "devastated" hung in the room for what seemed an eternity.

"We are going to be telling the boys tomorrow afternoon and a group of friends tomorrow evening. We ask that you not tell a soul, including your children, for twenty-four hours. Thank you again for being here with us. Are there any questions?"

"I don't know how something like this could happen," said my brother Brian, a highly regarded physician. He and his wife Beth were shaking their heads. "Doctors and nurses spend the better part of their days preventing tragedies like this."

"This is like an episode of *Dateline*," my brother Jeff said. His wife Carol looked like she wanted to punch him.

After Jeff's remark, Carolyn and I stood up and everyone else did the same.

Generally my family doesn't like to discuss tough topics, so I knew there would be very little talk after we were done. One by one, my siblings approached us as though we were standing next to a casket to offer their condolences, prayers, and support. I was very touched by my brother Aaron, my best man and the brother closest to me in age. He gripped me and said, "I am so proud of both of you." Each sibling left silently. After a few minutes the only three remaining were my mom and Carolyn and me. I embraced my mom. She was still shaken, but I knew my sisters Kelly and Patti would help her.

On the way home we were relieved and even laughed a little. My family's Irish Catholic heritage gives us special talents when it comes to bottling things up. We are there to support each other, but we avoid hugs and expressions of emotion.

"I bet when I started sobbing, everyone wanted to run from the room," Carolyn said.

"The support was tremendous, but seeing the family leave their emotional comfort zone was just so painful. We would rather do *anything* than have to share feelings," I said.

When we got home that evening, Carolyn's parents had waited up for us to make sure everything had gone all right. I doubt that anyone really slept well that night. We had a big day ahead. There would be Drew's race, and then we would have to tell the boys, and finally our friends.

After a restless night of sleep, we headed to Drew's school for a slight reprieve from the stress that was threatening to overwhelm this forty-eight-hour period. Before the race, 1,000 cheering alumni, students, and their families gathered near the starting line. I took a deep breath and inhaled the fresh spring air on a beautiful day. The doors of the school opened, and the 180 seventh- and eighth graders, wearing their neon-green race T-shirts, poured out onto the sidewalk, high-fiving and smiling as they jogged to the starting line. I caught Drew's eye and nodded to him. I knew he had been waiting years for this moment. I saw determination in him, and confidence. The horn sounded, and a herd of pumped-up teenagers took off. As Drew went by, I was so glad we had not broken the news to him and Ryan the night before. The run was tough enough.

I wasn't just rooting for Drew, though. I had coached many of these kids, and I wanted them all to do well. I jumped in my car and drove to a point about a mile into the route where I could cheer the runners on. Drew's stride was smooth and in control. This appeared to be Drew's day.

"Drew, looking strong! Keep it going! I'll see you at the finish line!"

At the finish line, I focused my video camera at the place where the kids would take the final turn. I was still worried about Drew. What if he cramped? What if he turned an ankle? He was running so well. I didn't want something like that to ruin this spectacular performance.

The lead bike came around the corner, and right behind him, I recognized Drew's stride. As Drew came more into focus, I pictured him running with me back in kindergarten. Nine years before, I'd had to slow down to run with him. Now I couldn't keep up with him. Drew was about 150 meters away. Then, before I knew it, he was upon me. I realized I needed to sprint to film him crossing the finish line.

As Drew broke the tape and the crowd cheered, a chill went up my spine. He had done it! I watched him working to catch his breath as he poured water on his head. I placed my arm on his shoulder.

"Drew, fantastic run. You earned this. Enjoy it."

For sixteen minutes I had put aside the pregnancy and reveled in Drew's run, but my reprieve was over. I was a proud dad. I had been robbed of a great deal of normal time with Drew, Ryan, and Mary Kate during the previous ninety days and would continue, it seemed, to miss a lot into the foreseeable future. I would be a fool to think this had not already hurt them. However, what was going to win this moment was a family celebration for Drew's huge accomplishment. The period after the race, when the kids were taking pictures of each other and congratulating one another, capped off a big week when everyone had done their best. It was a perfect moment to set aside the stresses of life, and that's what we did.

As the event was winding down, I walked to the car with Drew by my side and saw a young man who was coming into his own. Although he hated getting hugs, I gave one to him anyway and then made the drive back to work and reality. When the boys got home, it would be time to tell them the news.

We needed to keep ourselves as even-keeled as possible to make this go well for the boys. As a principal, Carolyn had seen many times how children suffering through a tragedy follow the emotional lead of their parents. If a mom ends up in the fetal position in the corner, her children mimic that response. But if a parent is rational, his or her children remain rational. We decided to be straightforward about what had happened, explain why we had decided to do what we were going to do, and then assure them that, although the whole thing was difficult, everything would be okay. Unlike the way we approached our other meetings, we didn't hold our outline as we spoke. This was parent to child, and we wanted to be open to what they had to say, not restricted by a list.

Both Drew and Ryan were in a great mood when they got home and looking forward to the weekend. Carolyn and I were waiting in the family room.

"Drew and Ryan, we need to talk to you about something. Please take a seat."

Their smiles faded as they sat down.

"We have some news to share with you," I said. "It is not good news, but we don't want you to worry. No one is sick or anything like that."

"You know how there are eleven years between Ryan and Mary Kate?" Carolyn said.

They nodded.

"Well, we didn't plan it that way. We love you guys so much, and we always wanted more kids, so after you were born, Ryan, we kept trying and trying to have more, but it never seemed to work out. We finally found a doctor who helped us get pregnant with your sister. Have you ever heard of in vitro fertilization?"

"Yup. That's what that lady did who got eight babies," Drew said, with a serious look of concern on his face.

"Well, that is what we did to get Mary Kate. During that process, we made more embryos than we could use. So we had them frozen so we could try again. We tried again a few months ago, but the doctor made a big mistake and put someone else's embryos inside of me."

From the look on the boys' faces, it wasn't clear that they really comprehended what had happened. I remembered how the disclosure had gone the day before: the news was so shocking that everyone we told needed to hear it twice.

"Mom is pregnant, but the baby doesn't belong to us," I said. "It belongs to another family, and they want him."

The boys were speechless.

"We met the other mom and dad last week, and they seemed very nice and were very grateful that we decided not to have an abortion," Carolyn continued. "They really want their baby."

"So, Mom is going to have the baby, and then we have to give him to his parents," I said again. "Do you understand?"

They both nodded. Ryan was looking straight ahead, but Drew was looking right at me.

"Do you have any questions?" I asked them.

They both hesitated, and then the firing began with Ryan.

"Do you have to give him back? I mean, wouldn't he like it here with our family?"

His question broke our hearts.

"Yes. I'm sure he would love it here with our family. But his genetic parents want him. It wouldn't be right for us to keep him."

"Are they nice people?" Drew asked. "Were they nice to you when you met them?"

"Yes. They were nice to us," I said. "They already have two kids, and they really want this one too."

"Does the other family go to church?" Ryan asked.

"Do they smoke?" Drew wanted to know. "What do they do for a living? Where do they live?"

I could see where their minds were going. We had it pretty good. We were a close-knit family. Wouldn't this baby just want to stay here?

"Who else knows?" Drew asked.

"Well, we told Grandma Kate, Grandma Linda, and Papa yesterday, and we told all of my family last night," I said. "We didn't want to tell you until after the 5K was over with. We knew it was going to be a big day for you, and we didn't want to distract you from your goals today."

Drew shook his head. He got it.

"At five this afternoon," I said, "we are leaving to go up to church. We called a meeting with all of our friends in one of the meeting rooms. We are going to tell them then."

Drew wanted to know who was going to be at that meeting. We reviewed the list with him, and he suggested a few additions, all parents of friends of his. This surprised us, but we made a few quick phone calls and got the parents he requested to agree to come.

"I knew you were pregnant," Drew confessed.

"You did? How?" Carolyn asked.

"You left that heartbeat thing on the floor next to the bed a couple of times. I figured you must be listening to the baby like you did with Mary Kate. I've known for three weeks."

"Oh, Drew, I feel so bad about that," Carolyn said. "You thought for weeks that you were going to get a little brother or sister. We probably shocked you more than we ever could have realized. Are you okay?"

He nodded his head yes. But I am not sure there was much conviction behind that answer. This would be tough for Drew, since he had already planned on another sibling.

"Are you going to sue?" Drew asked.

I didn't expect to get that kind of question from the boys.

"We have attorneys who are taking care of that part. Don't worry about that," I said.

"Well, I think you should sue. They shouldn't be allowed to make these kinds of mistakes. They should get in trouble for this."

I told him I agreed with him.

I looked at Ryan and saw sadness in his eyes as he looked out the window. He has a gift for compassion and loved being a great big brother and protector of Mary Kate, and I am sure he was seeing that opportunity vanish for this next child.

"Drew and Ryan, this is a difficult situation, and we are handling it the best we know how," I said. "There will be tough days ahead, but we will get through this as a family. If you have any questions at any time, please let us know. We love you very much, and trust me when I say we will be just fine."

We were so proud of our sons. They handled this news with a kind of maturity that was way beyond their years.

We shifted our attention to the last meeting in this series: with our friends. I hoped this would be the easiest. We were now pretty practiced at discussing the situation. Prior to departing for church, I went for a run to clear my head. For the first time in months the run helped me find release. Letting the secret go was like having shackles removed from my feet. The double life we had been leading was now coming to an end.

CAROLYN

To GIVE THE SYLVANIA grapevine as little time as possible to buzz, we didn't notify our friends about the five o'clock meeting until around noon. Sean again reassured everyone that no one was sick or dying, but that was about all he said.

Even though we gave them as little lead time as possible to talk among themselves, one of my dear friends became quite frantic upon learning of the get-together. Amny has been my friend for thirteen years, and she has always been in my loop of top-secret pregnancy information. The idea that something could be happening to me that she didn't know about made her panic. She called to insist that she was coming over immediately.

"You can't come over. I can't tell you anything yet."

"You are scaring me. I am coming over now."

"Amny, I can't let you do that. I know Sean told you that no one is dying, no one is sick. I can add that our marriage is fine, and that no one has done anything illegal. Stop trying to guess because you will never figure it out. It is not anything that has ever happened before, and because it is so upsetting to me, I don't want to explain it more than I have to. You have to wait, but it will be okay."

Amny was exasperated, but the only way to do this was as planned. She would just have to wait.

Amny wasn't the only one who freaked out upon receiving the call from Sean. By the time we arrived at church, our friends had dreamed up every horrid scenario under the sun. They had us divorcing, terminally ill, or leaving the Church. As if we would hold a meeting at church to announce that we were leaving the Church. No one came up with anything close to reality. I guess that speaks to how unbelievable our circumstances were.

When we got out of the car in the church parking lot, I grabbed Sean's "mega" binder and carried it into the meeting to cover my obviously protruding belly. I wore my new maternity top, a shirt that clearly showed I was pregnant. As we entered the room, a hush fell over the crowd.

We took our seats at the front of the room. Then I looked up and surveyed the men and women I cared deeply about in our town. These were the moms and dads we had worked with, grown up with, and sat with in the freezing snow at soccer games. They all had been to our house many times for beers and barbecues. Sean had coached almost all of their kids in one sport or another. There were members of my book club and prayer group in the room, and many of them worshiped with us every Sunday. I was so touched that they had all dropped everything—some of them even postponing trips out of town—to be with us at this moment.

Sean cut to the chase very quickly, as we had done in all of our other meetings. I was staring down, but looked up just as Sean was saying, "Another couple's embryos were transferred into Carolyn. She is pregnant with another couple's baby." My friend Shannon's eyes closed as if she was trying to make what he said go away. As if she could just open her eyes again and it would all be a bad dream.

I also caught the gobsmacked faces of my friends Kris and Katie. Kris had been someone to whom I reached out after my miscarriage in 2006. Her eyes and Katie's eyes immediately filled with tears. Kris was gripping the edge of her chair as if she was trying not to fall over. She was white-knuckled.

When it was my turn, I skipped the line about being devastated that had made me cry the night before and instead explained what would and wouldn't be helpful to us.

"I know you all are wondering what you can say to us to make us feel better. I don't have an answer for you. I guess it would be more comfortable if we could pretend that this was not happening. I don't want to be the elephant in the room . . . literally."

That got a laugh.

"Since I know you may not know what to say, I'm going to give you a few tips on what not to say."

Again, they all laughed.

"There are three things that well-intentioned people have already said to us that are not helpful. The first is this: 'God only gives you what you can handle.' I don't believe this. I have seen in my life many people who have landed in situations that they couldn't handle. I hope we are strong enough to handle this, but I will never accept this as a test from God. I don't think God tests people.

"Another one that gets to me is the idea that 'this is God's plan.' That theology doesn't work for us. We don't believe that God sits up in heaven and decides who gets what tragedy or blessing. We are certain that God didn't do this to us. We just know it happened, and now we are going to lean on our faith, and on you, to get through.

"The last thing that I would be happy to never hear again is: 'Something good will come of this.' I have no idea what is going to come of this, but I can confidently tell you that, regardless of how this turns out, we will never, ever look back on this event and say, 'Good thing that happened.'

"I hope I find the strength to get through this. I was inspired while listening to Jackie Frisch talk last night. She is so strong and full of grace. I am not where she is. Maybe someday I will be, but right now I'm not. I'm really going to need your help."

I finished my part and looked up for the second time in the meeting while Sean moved on. I noticed my friend Anne in the back of the room next to her husband Mike, with tears streaming down her face. I saw my friend Kathleen, who was clearly panic-stricken. I learned later she had missed the beginning of our talk and thought we had found out that Mary Kate wasn't ours and we were going to lose her. My friend Melanie quickly explained the situation to her. Kathleen burst into tears out of relief, until she finally understood the real problem. Then she was sobbing all over again.

Sean finished, and we asked if anyone had any questions, at which point my dear friend Rachel piped up. Rachel will say anything, so I braced myself.

"I sure hope you are going to sue the doctor responsible."

Leave it to Rachel to blurt out the question that I'm sure everyone else was thinking. Sean explained to her that we were going to keep that part of this private. There were a few more questions about how we were telling our kids, and we explained that we had told our kids the truth earlier that day.

"We're not going to tell you how to handle this with your children. That's your job as their parents. But if for any reason you decide not to tell your kids, please let us know. We'll do our best to stay away from them until the end of the pregnancy," Sean said.

With that, we stood up as the meeting felt complete.

"Well, I guess you are pregnant," Amny said.

We all chuckled.

"I just want you to know that I think what you are doing is awesome," our friend Jenny said. "You are saving this baby's life, and he is darn lucky he is where he is. I am proud to call you my friends."

Everyone kind of "hear-hear-ed," and I choked up.

The meeting had gone perfectly as planned. Until we went to leave.

One thing everyone should know about Sean is that he is not a man-hugger. Sean will gladly kiss and hug any woman around, but when it comes to showing affection to men, a firm handshake does him just fine. As people stood up to leave, we were surprised that everyone lined up to express their condolences, just like Sean's siblings had. There were lots of tears, and there were hugs for me, and of course Sean was lapping up the affection from my girlfriends, since they are not a bad bunch to look at. However, there were some awkward moments when Sean didn't know what to do with the men. Handshake or man-hug? By the time it was over, Sean was sweating.

"You okay?" I asked as we got in the car to go home.

"Yeah . . . but I could have done without the hugging. I didn't know what to do. Is he leaning in to pat me on the back? Do we hug? Uncomfortable."

I burst out laughing. I guess I should have added to my little speech on what not to say that Sean would not be hugging any men tonight, so don't try.

We laughed on the way home. We were relieved. Our secret was really out, and we hoped we would now get the support we yearned for.

CHAPTER 12

The Elephant in the Room

CAROLYN

IN THE WEEKS AFTER we met the Morells and told everyone of our troubles, Sean and I decided it was stupid to continue communicating with them through attorneys. They seemed nice enough and were very respectful of us during our meeting. We needed to get to know each other, to trust each other, and to find a way, I hoped, to support each other through this. If we could pull that together, then we'd have an easier time staying close after the baby was born.

Although I was warming to Shannon, I couldn't forget the effect that her first letter had had on me. To keep communication with her from leaking into my everyday business, I created a new e-mail address that I gave only to her. That way, I could open that e-mail account only when I was mentally prepared to receive a message from her. Shannon was happy to get my e-mail and phone numbers. She was enthusiastic about any sign that I would allow her a closer view of the pregnancy. The morning before I was scheduled to have the amniocentesis test, I sent Shannon an e-mail letting her know when the test was happening and invited her to call me that night to check on how the procedure went.

Sean and I met at the lab half an hour before the test so that we would have plenty of time to fill out the paperwork. When I entered the maternal fetal medicine waiting room, the receptionist handed me a clipboard, a pen, and a stack of forms to complete.

"Here. You do your part," I said, handing Sean a stack of papers. For this test, he was considered the birth father, which meant that he had to sign numerous waivers promising not to sue if the procedure went poorly.

As he started filling out his forms, I studied my questionnaire.

"I can't fill this out. Look at these questions," I said.

The first question was the age of the mother at the time of conception, then the age of the father, and the health history of the baby's genetic relatives. I flipped page after page to see whether I knew the answers to any of the questions.

"The only thing I know is Shannon's age at the time of her original IVF. That's it. I can't answer a single question."

"Carolyn Savage?"

We followed a nurse into a consult office.

"Wait right here for Jenny. She'll be with you in a moment."

I wondered who Jenny was until I noticed the framed degrees hanging on the wall.

"Oh, man. This is the office of the genetic counselor."

Before Sean could react, Jenny bounced into her office and took her seat at the desk.

"Hi there. I'm here to talk to you about the genetic test results that you will be receiving about your baby in a few weeks. Can I see your paperwork?"

Begrudgingly, I slid the incomplete questionnaire toward her.

"Didn't you have time to fill it out?"

"Uh . . . no. We can't fill it out. We don't have that kind of information about the genetic history of my baby." I was annoyed. The doctor who was performing the amnio knew about our situation, and I explained it to the nurse before I ordered the DNA diagnostic kit. Why didn't Jenny know?

Suddenly a lightbulb went off in Jenny's head.

"Oh. This is an anonymous embryo donation?"

For crying out loud. No one had told this woman why we were there.

"No. I'm pregnant as a result of a botched IVF. My doctor transferred the wrong embryos into me. We need to confirm genetic parentage with our amnio."

Jenny was stupefied.

"I didn't know that could happen. Did it happen in this fertility clinic?" she said.

"No. It didn't happen here. Please be clear on that."

She looked relieved. "If the baby is confirmed not to be yours, are you going to terminate?"

"No. We're going to keep the pregnancy," I said impatiently. "We need to make sure that the baby truly isn't ours and that the people they think he belongs to are really his genetic family. We don't want to give the baby away if we don't have to. And we certainly need to make sure that if we have to, we give the baby to the right people!"

I was stressed enough. I didn't need to get even more upset by having to explain this.

"You know, it seems that we don't need to meet with you," I said. "So, can we just go back to the waiting room?"

"Yes, but first let me explain the procedure," she said. "You'll lie down on the table. They will date the baby's gestational age via ultrasound, then identify a safe area in which to place the catheter that will draw up the amniotic fluid. The whole thing will last less than a minute."

"We're ready for you," said a nurse, addressing us from the doorway to the examining rooms. She escorted us to the room where I lay down on an ultrasound table. Sean sat in a chair nearby and pulled out his planner to review his schedule for the rest of the day. Sean hates medical stuff. He had brought a bag full of work, expecting that there would be a lot of time to pass. The doctor entered and introduced himself.

"Hi. I'll be doing the amnio today, and Chris here will be handling the ultrasound," the doctor said as Chris squirted ultrasound gel on my belly.

"Now, I'm in the camp of not numbing my patients before amnios. I figure by the time I'm done poking you with all of the numbing medications, I might as well have just done the amnio," the doctor quickly explained.

Holy Moly. No numbing medication? What do you mean it is just as painful as the numbing meds? How many amnios have you had, buddy?

"Okay, are we ready? Now, you may feel some pressure, but this will only take a minute."

He was holding a metal thingamajigger that looked like a knitting needle.

Seriously? You are going to stab me and my baby with that? I can't believe women actually consent to this voluntarily.

My first instinct was to jump from the table and run from the room. Before I could flee, he plunged the needle into my abdomen, through my uterine wall, and pierced my amniotic sac.

I gasped as my uterus contracted and pain shot out of my cervix. I couldn't breathe. This was definitely taking longer than a minute.

"Now, we have to draw up more fluid than normal because of the extra paternity testing," he said as he started to fill a second vial.

Please be over. Please be over. What if this hurts the baby? What if our need to know ends this pregnancy?

"Okay. All through," he said as he withdrew the catheter and I took a deep breath. "No leakage. Looks good."

I looked over at a pale-faced Sean, who looked like he was the one who'd just had the amnio.

"Now, Chris will finish a more thorough ultrasound, and then a nurse will come in to complete the DNA kit information with you. Nice meeting you," he said and exited.

Chris spent about five more minutes taking measurements of the baby.

"Do you know what you are having yet?"

"No. Can you tell?"

"Looks like a boy to me." She moved the wand a little more. "Yup. Definitely a boy."

And I smiled. My Little One was a Little Man! A son.

A few minutes later, the nurse swabbed inside our cheeks to collect DNA samples.

"Now, you take it easy the rest of the day," she told me. She handed me discharge instructions. "You can resume normal activities tomorrow. Call us if you have any of these symptoms."

Back home, I went straight to bed. That evening, still resting, I recognized the Morells' number before I answered the phone.

"Hi, Shannon. Everything went well. I'm resting, and there was no leaking or bleeding afterwards. I'm staying off my feet until tomorrow to be safe."

"How was it? I never had an amnio with the girls."

"It was awful. I had no idea it was that painful. I would never, ever do that test if we hadn't been put in this position. Hey, the ultrasound person today thinks it is a boy."

"Oh. Do you think the tech was right? I mean, we already have two girls and all this girl stuff. A boy would be nice, but really different. I grew up with a sister. No brothers. So . . . a boy. Wow, that would be different."

"I don't know if she was right. I think we'll know more when we get a definitive answer from the genetic testing in a few weeks."

"Okay. I just have so much girl stuff. And this baby will be born in the same season as my twins. So their clothes will fit perfect and I've saved everything. But if it is a boy, I guess I can sell all the girly things in a garage sale and add boy toys. If it's a boy, we'll have to move the girls' rooms around. Right now, they have their own bedrooms, but we can't put a boy in with a girl. So I'll have to put the twins together and repaint a room so it is more little boy."

"Uh-huh. I wanted to let you know that we told our family and friends last week."

"How did they take it?"

"Well, it was hard. Everyone was extremely supportive, but it is all very awkward."

"Yeah. That's the way it's going to be for us when we bring the baby home. Awkward. We just don't know what to tell people. I wanted to keep our use of IVF private. I don't know how to do that and explain where this baby came from. I'm thinking we could tell everyone we used a surrogate. That is closest to the truth. This is like a surrogacy."

"Oh. Okay. Well, I'm sure you'll do what you think is best for your family."

"Yeah. We are just very private people. I don't want people at work to know my business. You know?"

"I can only imagine how difficult this is for you," I said.

"And I'm afraid of what people are going to say. The other day I confided in our pediatrician what happened, and he said, 'And you think that baby is yours?' This caught me completely off-guard. I told him that they were our embryos. He said, 'An embryo is just a few cells. A woman turns them into a baby.' Can you believe he thinks that?"

"I can't believe that he thinks this baby doesn't legally belong to you."

"I'm afraid that that's what people are going to think, that the baby really belongs to you because your body carried it. I think people are not going to understand why we think he is ours. You know?"

"Legally, he is yours shortly after delivery. So what people think, what your pediatrician thinks, doesn't matter."

"Yeah. I just don't think people will understand our loss. How we are missing his pregnancy. I don't get to experience this with my girls. I was looking forward to being pregnant again. I'll never feel him kick. I don't get to love him the way I loved my girls before they were born."

I knew she was feeling cheated, and I understood why. I was the wrong person to ask for sympathy, though.

SEAN

WE WERE FLOODED WITH SUPPORT from the moment we told people our news. In addition to Marty, my closest high school friends, Craig Bruning, Greg Periatt, and Matt Dzierwa, had been fiercely loyal through the years. I knew they would be there. We had been friends for over twenty-five years and lived through the highs and lows of life supporting each other. They, along with my friends Dan, Steve, and Tony, formed an immediate support system for me. The calls kept coming that night and throughout the weekend. On Sunday my brother Kevin stopped by without notice. Kevin had been out of town and missed our family meeting. His wife JoAnn had filled him in, and on his way back into town he came straight to our house. As we reviewed the details of the situation with him, I let a call from my uncle Bob go to voice mail. Uncle Bob, who was my father's business partner, was quite emotional. When I listened to his voice-mail message, I heard him sobbing, with a few words mixed in. I would be sitting down with the partners of Savage & Associates, Dan, Tim, Phil, and Mark, the next day. The shock wave was spreading, and the initial support was gratifying.

Then soon, our phone quit ringing. The invitations to join other families at their houses for dinner or a backyard barbecue dried up. Gradually it dawned on us that, despite the fact that our friends' hearts were open to us and we were certainly in their prayers, no one knew quite what to say. Maybe our friends were frightened of saying the wrong thing. How were they to know what we were feeling on any particular day?

I understood that hesitation. I never knew where Carolyn would be emotionally when I got a call from her or when I got home. I might find her happy because the baby was very active, or I might find her deep in sorrow for the very same reason. Still, the fact that many of our friends kept to themselves hurt. On the other hand, I am not sure there were many events to which we would have accepted invitations. Part of the problem was that, while others were distancing themselves, we were also withdrawing. We were sick of people's sympathetic looks and their stares.

Carolyn was having tough weeks physically too. The "morning" sickness hit her almost every night, and she was on anti-nausea medication that made her sleepy. She was resting a great deal and had low energy when she was awake. Many days she was crabby and down, depleted. Did we want to show this face to the world? Self-pity is not our game, especially in public. Did we privately feel bad for ourselves? Yes. Do people really want to hear someone else cry about their situation? No. So while we had decided that it was time to share our secret with the world, it turned out that our world was not quite ready to jump into the fire with us—and we weren't quite ready to invite them.

As a result, we decided to change our Sunday routine. Even though St. Joe's has five masses each weekend, we had always attended the same one every week. By May, Carolyn and I were attending church separately, and we did not sit in our normal spots. On Sunday mornings, while the boys and I slept late, Carolyn slipped out of bed at 6:45. She and Mary Kate attended 7:30 mass seated in the cry room, the soundproof room the church maintained for parents with noisy babies. Most of the regulars at that early morning mass were senior citizens. Carolyn was isolated and unnoticed.

Around 9:30, I'd get the boys up and out the door for 10:30 mass. We would leave the house just in time to arrive when mass began. Catholic churches have "unassigned" assigned seating. The Savages' spot in our church was north side, front row, seats 1–5, for 10:30 mass. There the boys would open the doors for the assisted-living parishioners who left after communion. Another reason we chose that spot was to make sure the kids paid attention. No room for screwing around in the front row. Not only was God watching, but the priest was as well.

Arriving as late as we did, the boys and I now stood at the back, leaning up against the wall, and we bolted as soon as mass was over so I could get back and help Carolyn with Mary Kate and avoid awkward post-mass conversations. An unintended result of this new routine was that we fell off most of our friends' radar. We weren't around for those moments afterward when families spontaneously agreed to get together for cookouts or made plans for the upcoming week.

Our withdrawal from church, however, was about more than just our discomfort being around others. Deep down, I was concerned about how the Catholic Church would react to our situation. Father Cardone, our pastor Father Dennis Metzger, and our very close family friend Father Richard Wurzel were there when we needed them, but how the hierarchy of the Church was going to treat us was an unknown, and my gut was telling me it wasn't going to be good. I was angry at the thought that at the end of this my church probably would not be there to lift us up, so I moved from sitting right up front to leaning up against the back wall. What a rebel!

All of this change unmoored me. As a result, nighttime quickly became my enemy. During periods of enormous stress, I don't sleep well. Twelve years ago, when Ryan came home from the hospital, he slept in a small crib next to our bed hooked to a breathing monitor. I regularly woke up in a panic believing that he was in our bed and I had rolled on top of him. This crisis brought back my crazy sleep patterns. I often woke up to the sound of Carolyn's panicked voice.

"Sean! Sean! What are you doing?"

I would find myself standing in a part of our bedroom far away from the bed. Back in bed, I'd drift to sleep, only to return to a nightmare about losing a baby. I'd wake up with sweat dripping down my forehead. Gradually, I found that I was starting my work-day at 4:00 A.M. Better for me to live a nightmare than dream one.

The other layer of this problem was how to talk to people who didn't know. Once we disclosed our situation and Carolyn started wearing maternity clothes, even strangers congratulated the lucky mom. We didn't know how to respond. We had no idea how much these strangers or acquaintances knew. We also were unsure how much the story was getting distorted by being passed down the grapevine. We felt uneasy telling a partial truth in front of an au-dience that included people who knew the full story. As a result, Carolyn felt that all eyes were on her everywhere she went, particu-larly at the park, where her pregnancy was a prominent subject of conversation among the mothers.

"Wow. You're having another one?" one woman said to Caro-lyn while we were at the swings with MK, who was quite petite for her age. "You're going to have your hands full!"

I could see Carolyn mentally running through the criteria for deciding whether to explain. Did she know this person on a first-name basis? Would she see her again after the baby was born and gone? In this case, the answer was yes to both questions, so Carolyn proceeded with what she called her "bombshell in a nutshell."

"Well, it's not what you think," Carolyn said. The woman looked stricken, as if she'd just committed one of the world's most feared faux pas—insinuating that a woman is pregnant when she is really not!

"I am pregnant, but you see, Mary Kate was an IVF baby, and when we did her IVF cycle we froze the embryos we didn't use. We went back to our doctor this past February to try to transfer our own embryos that had been frozen, but he made a mistake and

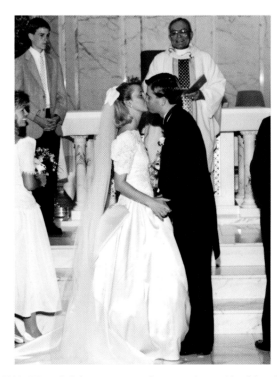

May 29, 1993: We sealed the sacrament of our marriage with a kiss while Father Richard Wurzel looked on, as well as Carolyn's maid of honor, Laura Radtke-Daly.

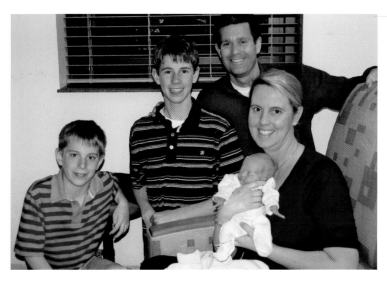

April 16, 2008: We were all smiles as the boys got to meet their baby sister for the first time in the NICU of Mercy St. Vincent Medical Center.

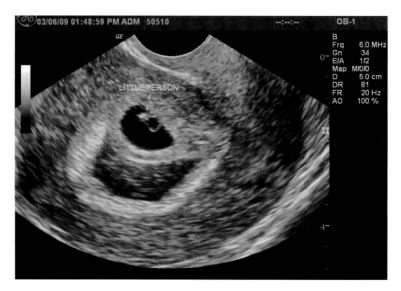

Logan's third ultrasound picture, taken only one week after his heart
started beating.

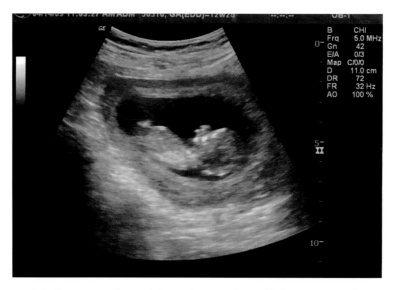

Baby Logan at twelve weeks' gestation, complete with fingers, toes, and a
heart that was strong and growing!

In late May 2009, the error was confirmed through DNA testing of Carolyn's amniotic fluid obtained during an amniocentesis. The results we received from DNA Diagnostics Center indicated that Carolyn had zero genetic connection to the baby she was carrying. Sean received identical results the same day.

DNA Test Report

DDC is accredited/certified by AABB, CAP, ACLASS-International, ISO/IEC 17025, CLIA, NYSDOH & ASCLD/LAB-International.

Case: 358803		Alleged MOTHER		CHILD	
Name		Carolyn J. Savage		Amniocentesis	
Race		Caucasian			
Date Collected		5/12/2009		5/12/2009	
Test No.		358803-10		358803-20	
Locus	MI	Allele Sizes		Allele Sizes	
D8S1179	1.99	13	14	13	14
D21S11	4.47	29	31	29	31
D7S820	0.00	8	14	9	10
CSF1PO	1.61	11	12	11	12
D3S1358	1.95	15	16	15	16
TH01	0.00	9.3	10	7	9
D13S317	0.00	8	13	11	
D16S539	1.41	11	13	9	13
D2S1338	0.00	19	23	20	24
D19S433	2.05	14	15	14	15
vWA	0.00	14	17	16	18
TPOX	1.86	8		8	
D18S51	0.00	16	17	12	13
D5S818	0.00	11		12	13
FGA	0.00	20	24	22	23

Interpretation: RN. 193192

Combined Maternity Index: **0**   Probability of Maternity: **0**%

The alleged mother is excluded as the biological mother of the prenatal sample. This conclusion is based on the non-matching alleles observed at the loci listed above with a MI equal to 0. The alleged mother lacks the genetic markers that must be contributed to the child by the biological mother. The probability of maternity is 0%.

Subscribed and sworn before me on May 19, 2009

Jennie A. Roberts
Notary Public, State of Ohio
My Commission Expires December 29, 2009

I, the undersigned, verify that the interpretation of the results is correct as reported on 5/19/2009

Melissa D. Kahsar

Michael L. Baird, Ph.D.   Thomas M. Reid, Ph.D.
Melissa D. Kahsar, Ph.D.   Keen A. Wilson, Ph.D.
L. Farris Hanna, Ph.D.   Pierig Lepont, Ph.D.
Marco Scarpetta, Ph.D.   Julie A. Heinig, Ph.D.

+1-513-881-7800   One DDC Way, Fairfield, OH 45014   U.S.A.   DNACenter.com

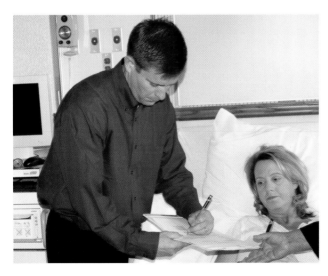

September 25, 2009: Sean signing legal documents relinquishing custody of Logan to Paul and Shannon Morell.

COURT OF COMMON PLEAS OF LUCAS COUNTY, OHIO
JUVENILE DIVISION

In Re: Male Infant Morell : CASE NO.
   a.k.a. Male Infant Savage :
   DOB: September 24, 2009 : JUDGE CONNIE ZEMMELMAN
             :

Paul Morell :
Shannon Morell :
             :
Complainants :
             :
vs. :
             :
Sean Savage. :
Carolyn Savage. : **AFFIDAVIT OF STIPULATED FACTS**
             :
Respondents :

> FILED
> Juvenile Division
> CLERK'S OFFICE
>
> SEP 25 2009
>
> Lucas Co. Com. Pleas Court
> #18

The Complainants and Respondents agree to the following facts:

1. Complainants Paul Morell and Shannon Morell are husband and wife.

2. Respondents Carolyn Savage and Sean Savage are husband and wife.

3. The parties submit themselves to the jurisdiction/venue of the Lucas County Common Pleas Court, Juvenile Division.

4. The child in question ("Child") was born on September 24, 2009 at St. Vincent Mercy Medical Center.

5. Because of an error by the IVF laboratory, and confirmed by genetic testing, Carolyn Savage and Sean Savage are not genetically related to the child gestated by Carolyn Savage. Pursuant to genetic testing and based on information and belief, Paul Morell and Shannon Morell are the biological parents of said Child.

6. Complainants desire parental rights to said Child. Respondents do not desire parental rights to said Child.

7. Respondents desire and intend to sever all legal ties with said Child with respect to inheritance, custody or any other parental right.

8. The parties agree that there exists a parent/child relationship between the Child and the Complainants.

_____
Sean Savage

_____
Carolyn Savage

STATE OF OHIO, COUNTY OF LUCAS, SS:

Before me, a Notary in and for said County, personally appeared the above named Carolyn Savage and Sean Savage who acknowledge that they did sign this instrument and the same is their voluntary act and deed.

IN TESTIMONY WHEREOF, I have hereunto subscribed my name and affixed my official seal this _____ day of September, 2009.

_____
Notary Public

_____
Paul Morell

_____
Shannon Morell

STATE OF OHIO, COUNTY OF LUCAS, SS:

Before me, a Notary in and for said County, personally appeared the above named Paul Morell and Shannon Morell who acknowledge that they did sign this instrument and the same is their voluntary act and deed.

IN TESTIMONY WHEREOF, I have hereunto subscribed my name and affixed my official seal this _____ day of September, 2009.

_____
Notary Public

_____
Ellen Essig (0037344)
Attorney for Complainants
Katz, Greenberger & Norton LLP
105 E. Fourth St., Ste. 400
Cincinnati, Ohio 45202
(513) 698-9345

_____
Mary Smith (0030530)
Attorney for Respondents
1200 Edison Plaza
300 Madison Avenue
Toledo, Ohio 43604-1556
(419) 243-6281

255800

The court documents completed on September 25, 2009, giving full custody to Paul and Shannon Morell less than twenty-four hours after Carolyn gave birth to Logan.

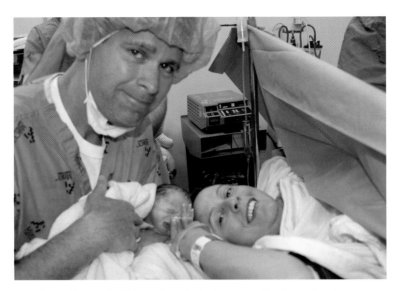

September 24, 2009: Sean introducing Logan to Carolyn only minutes after his birth.

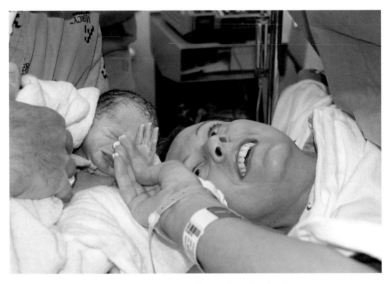

Logan and Carolyn meeting face to face for the first time.

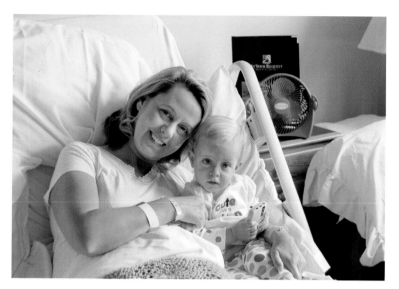

September 25, 2009: Mary Kate visiting her mommy in the hospital
the day after Logan was born.

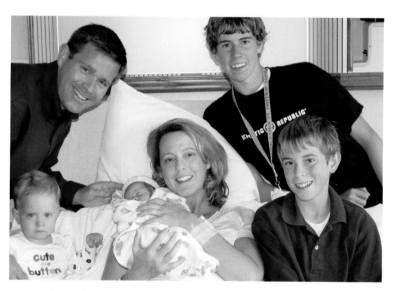

September 25, 2009: Our family of six, if only for a few minutes.

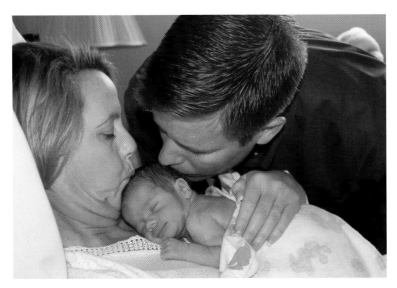

September 25, 2009: Loving on our precious baby Logan before he left
to go home with Paul and Shannon Morell.

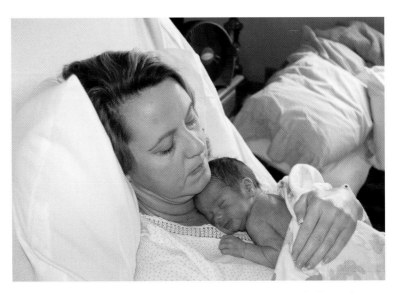

September 25, 2009: Peace. Our one and only snuggle in the hospital.

put the wrong embryos inside of me. I am pregnant with the wrong baby and will lose him upon delivery."

Then she paused.

"Don't worry. We are doing okay. I'm sorry. Are you okay?"

The woman was so shaken that Carolyn ended up consoling her through the shock and then accepting her condolences. It was encounters like this one that just made it easier to stay home.

The other thing that surprised us was how well the secret stayed contained among our friends. I had assumed that within a few weeks of revealing the information the story would have made its way to the press and we'd be fielding calls from reporters. As we got further into the month of May, we breathed a sigh of relief and felt like we'd been blessed. Just in case, Carolyn and I spent an afternoon working on a statement to release requesting that reporters respect our privacy.

But we knew there was one event we couldn't miss: Festirama, the annual parish festival that begins Friday evening and ends Sunday evening. The church rents carnival rides and puts out a large food spread, erects a gambling tent, and sells beer for the adults. Carolyn and I always worked the fast-food tent for four hours Saturday evening, and I worked the basketball shooting game on Friday. Normally, I'm grinning from ear to ear when I take my shift at the basketball shoot, joking around and telling stories. This year I felt like hiding, and in fact I did hide in a way—behind a fake smile. Yet I knew I had to fulfill my obligation to the church. In normal times I enjoyed giving my time to the church, and even though we were hurting, I felt strongly that we needed to be there.

Upon arriving that Friday evening, the boys scattered as far as they could from Mom and Dad as quickly as possible. Carolyn and I couldn't walk ten feet without seeing someone we knew. We were acutely aware of the unanswerable question echoing in our heads, *What do they know?*

Carolyn eventually accompanied one of her close friends to the

fast-food tent to sit down and talk at a table. I decided to keep cir-
culating. As I walked around with Mary Kate in a stroller, I ran into
Mike, a good buddy of mine from high school. I wasn't in regular
touch with him, so he was not one of those we had invited to the
meeting to tell our friends our news. "Mike! How are you doing?
How's the family?" I asked, genuinely happy to run into him. I
looked carefully at the expression on his face, trying to determine
whether he knew about our troubles.

"Great! We're all doing just great!" he said. "I saw Drew and
Ryan just a few minutes ago. Amazing how much they've grown.
Where's Carolyn? I haven't seen her tonight. How's everyone
doing?"

I was listening like a lawyer at a deposition for that slight change
in tone that would let me know that he was holding something back.
If he knew, the inflection in the question "How are you doing?"
would be knowing, even a little somber. I couldn't hear a hint of
that. But it suddenly didn't feel right to let it slide with someone I
had known for so long. At some point, probably even that weekend,
he would be in a conversation in which it would come up. If I let
it go and didn't tell him our news, he might feel slighted. So, to
escape the glare of the flashing neon lights and the chaos of the kids
running around, I pulled him aside. It was awkward for both of us.
I tried to calculate how many more people I would need to explain
this to.

The stress got to me, so I spent less time at Festirama that year
than I ever have, as did Carolyn. One can feel awkward only for so
long before needing to seek shelter from it.

While I was working my shift at the basketball shoot, it hit me
that life right then was nothing more than a grind. I had now just a
couple of places of refuge. One of those was home, where Carolyn
and I could be blunt.

And I could escape in coaching, where I focused completely
on the team. That spring at championships, Ryan turned in the

third-best time for a runner in his age group ever in the Diocese of Toledo. I could tell that he was doing great and that his best days as an athlete were still ahead. Drew registered CYO championships in the 1600 and 800. As I stood along the fence in each race and they came up the final stretch of the track, I had goose bumps of pride in my boys. After each race, when I went up to Drew and Ryan and congratulated them on their amazing performances, it probably meant more to me than it did to them. Searching for any bit of evidence that things were the same for our family, that we had shielded the boys from this mess, I took their success to be a good indicator.

I also took solace from knowing we would soon be on a trip to Florida that would offer us a needed break. I had a conference to attend there that would allow me to bring Carolyn and the boys. The couples who were coming from work already knew our situation. And we didn't have to tell those from other firms who didn't know. Carolyn and I were looking forward to leaving behind the complexities of home and relaxing for a few days.

CAROLYN

As we packed for Florida, I was happy we were going to get away from the prying eyes and whispered remarks of our small town. Among the couples from Savage & Associates on this trip was Sean's coworker Dan and his wife, my good friend Linda. Linda is my Jewish sister. Really, she's more like my Jewish mother, but she's not nearly old enough to be my mom, so sister fits. Linda was easy to talk to and never minded listening to me moan and groan about my life. I appreciated that she didn't tell me to look on the bright side. As soon as I told her about my pregnancy, she quickly became my "go-to" girl. She always gave me the blunt truth, with no sugarcoating and no attempts to avoid the subject. We both agreed that my situation "sucked." Plus, with Linda, I could laugh.

The last night of the trip was a formal dinner that the boys were happy didn't include them. They were old enough to fend for themselves and were hoping to take a trip over to the Magic Kingdom. It seemed like only yesterday that we were riding the Tea Cups with them and pushing them around Epcot in strollers. *I want to go with them*, I thought. A night in the amusement park sounded much better than a cocktail hour and dinner with people we barely knew. Savage & Associates wasn't the only firm invited to this event. I pulled out my black maternity wrap dress and squeezed my tired feet into my heels anyway.

Luckily, as we entered the ballroom of the Grand Floridian, I spotted Linda immediately.

"Thank God you're here. Do we have a table?"

"Yes. We'll all sit together." Linda had tipped the chairs of a table for eight, reserving it for us, in the corner of the ballroom.

"I need a drink!" she said.

"So do I," I joked.

Linda rolled her eyes.

"I'll have one for you," she said.

After she got her wine, we joined Dan and Sean, who were talking with some couples we didn't know. As I stood sipping my water, staring at the floor, the topic of conversation turned to my pregnancy.

"Congratulations. What number is this?"

I had no idea who this person was, so no explanation was required.

"Number four." I smiled.

"Oh. We have four too. How old are your other children?"

"Fourteen, twelve, and sixteen months."

"Oh my. Boys, girls?"

"Two boys and a girl."

"Do you know what this one is?"

"A boy."

"Oh, a third son. That's what I have! Boy, boy, girl, boy! You are going to love having a little guy full of energy running around. I bet his big brothers are excited."

"Yes."

Oh, how badly I wanted Drew and Ryan to celebrate the birth of a little brother and Mary Kate to have a playmate for life. With the birth of this baby, I would be reaching my lifelong goal of becoming a mother of four. I momentarily basked in my happiness. That only lasted for a few seconds before reality crept back in.

"Does your daughter understand that a new baby is coming?" the woman continued, shaking me out of my daydream.

"No. She has no idea. She just thinks Mama has a bump for her to sit on when I haul her around."

We all laughed because that was true. MK had developed a perch on top of this little guy. I think she thought he was a built-in bench.

"Will this be your last? Do you think you'll be done after this?"

I could hardly believe I was navigating the conversation. It was absurd to think that I was pretending to be excited about a pregnancy that was ripping my heart out. Linda quickly saved me.

"So what parks have you been too?"

And with that, the conversation took an appreciated turn. I glanced at Linda, who was rapid-firing questions at this woman to keep her from getting back to my pregnancy. I decided it would be best to excuse myself and go to the bathroom.

I opened the door to the handicapped stall, grabbed a paper toilet shield to protect my dress, attached it to the seat, and sat down.

Don't cry. You'll mess up your makeup. Stop it.

But it was too late. I grabbed a square of toilet paper to sop up my tears before my mascara started to run. I could hear the host ringing the bells indicating that guests should move to the ballroom for dinner. I took a few deep breaths and stared at my knees.

You are pathetic. Here you are, all dressed up, hiding in a bathroom stall, sitting on a toilet, your knees in your face, in the Happiest Place on Earth. Get a grip.

The women's room door opened.

"Carolyn? Are you in here?"

It was Linda.

"Yeah, I'm here." I stood up, pretending to finish my business by flushing the toilet, and came out of the stall.

"Are you all right?"

"Yes," I said as I washed my hands. "I'm fine. Now you know why I don't go out anymore. I can't do that day in and day out."

"I get it. You did fine."

I took a deep breath, and we left the bathroom together, her hand on my back comforting me in a gesture of sympathy and pushing me in an attempt to make me face my life.

CHAPTER 13

Turning Toward Hope

CAROLYN

MY LITTLE MAN WAS a mover and a shaker, a person who was sure to make his way through the world no matter what blocked his path. I didn't remember any of my other babies moving as much as this little guy. I would wake up in the morning, in those precious moments when my mind is opening up to the day, and feel him wriggling his way around, struggling to get free. I'd smile at the idea of him crawling down our hallway to his next adventure and finding something that caught his interest: a color, a shape, a sliver of light on a vase. That was the agony as we passed the halfway point in this pregnancy. Little Man was real to me, and every time I pictured him I could only see him in my arms or in our house tussling over a toy with Mary Kate. Every time I allowed myself to open to those happy ideas that sunny scene would end with a stab of despair.

He will not be toddling through your playroom, Carolyn. Stop this right now!

Yet I couldn't stop. How often had I pictured our family of four children? He just seemed to fit here. Throughout my years of infertility, I'd had a recurring dream of being nine months pregnant and driving to the hospital to deliver the baby. In that dream I was happy, excited. Then I'd wake and think, *Damn, it was just a dream*. As the pregnancy progressed with Little Man, that dream came more frequently. Only this time, when I woke from it, I actually was pregnant. As the baby became more real to me, the horror of the delivery room scenario terrified me. I simply couldn't think about it without tears.

For reasons I cannot explain, over and over again during the pregnancy I'd feel hope and joy yet seconds later find myself in the depths of sorrow. Several times a day I was swinging on this pendulum, as I had been when speaking to that woman at the party that night in Florida. My yearning for another child was so deep that the merest suggestion that my being pregnant was going to lead to this joyous event instantly set off happy thoughts and anticipation. Then I'd swing back the other direction on the pendulum, chiding myself for indulging that joy. As we came to the close of the second trimester, that despair was deeper than anything I'd ever felt.

My last shred of hope hung on the results of the DNA test. If the lab was so screwed up that it transferred the wrong embryo into me, there was a chance that its paperwork was off too, or that the way it filed the embryos was a jumble. Maybe when I got the DNA results I'd learn that these months of agony were misplaced emotions and this baby was really ours.

Finally the day arrived when the lab results appeared in the mailbox. I opened the unmarked envelope eagerly, unfolded the single piece of paper, and immediately directed my attention to the bottom line, where the numbers revealed the stark truth. There was 0 percent chance that this baby was ours. Not even 1 percent. I thought surely a little bit of my soul had crept into him. But I guess the DNA test couldn't measure my contribution.

I folded the test, shoved it into my purse, and turned my attention to the wonderful distraction I had that day: buying Drew a suit for his eighth-grade graduation. My feelings were all mixed up as we fitted my growing boy, my young man, for his first real adult garment. We found a sleek black suit with pinstripes. The coat fit well, but the pants needed to be altered because our ungainly son had a 27-inch waist and a 32-inch inseam. We had to special-order his dress shirt because he was a 14.5 neck with long arms, and he also needed dress shoes because he wore an 11, meaning he couldn't borrow Sean's size 9s. I reveled in pride as the tailor pinned his pants, thinking what a handsome young man Drew had become.

When we got home, I was planning to call Shannon to discuss the test results. What I didn't know was that the lab had also sent the results to the Morells, since Paul was tested as a probable DNA father. That night when the phone rang I saw that it was Shannon on the line.

"Well, the baby is ours! There's no doubt about it now," she said joyfully. "I guess you were right in insisting we do this. It is better to know."

"Yes," I said weakly. I had to be careful with my voice.

"You know, we didn't want to do this test. We didn't do an amnio with the twins. The risk was too great."

"I know. We never did an amnio before either. This is a different situation, of course," I said.

"Paul didn't like doing the test. The whole thing felt creepy," Shannon continued. "The lab he had to go to was in an unmarked office, and something about it made him feel like he was sneaking in through a back door."

"Oh, I'm sorry he was uncomfortable doing this," I said flatly. "I'm sorry he had to go through this."

I'm sorry I have to go through this too. I wondered if I should tell her how I was really feeling. I knew I couldn't speak up without falling apart, and I didn't think that would benefit either of us. If I cried, she might tell others that I was emotionally unstable, "a mess." Or she might worry that I was having second thoughts about keeping the baby. Most important, if I cried, I might cause her to feel guilty. I knew she was struggling. I didn't want to make her feel worse than she already did. That would be cruel. Nope, I had to stay quiet.

I ended the conversation by agreeing that I would undergo a 3-D ultrasound at twenty weeks so that Shannon and Paul could get a good look at the baby. I was dreading this event. We knew from my pregnancy with Mary Kate how vivid those images were. I wouldn't be with Linda at Dr. Read's office because they don't have the right kind of equipment for 3-D imaging. I was glad that Sean would be with me for this ordeal.

Before I knew it, the day for the ultrasound was upon us, and as we entered the exam room I was struck by how dark it was and how it lacked the cheerful atmosphere of Linda's "office." I positioned myself on the table with a feeling of dread. There was a part of me that didn't want to look at the screen, but I knew I would be unable to look away.

The technician spread the ultrasound gel across my belly, and before I could get too upset, up popped a perfect baby boy.

The tech was in a very sunny mood. She obviously loved giving happy parents a close-up of the baby they would soon hold in their arms.

"It's a boy!" she said cheerfully, manipulating the wand to give us a glimpse of all of his dimensions. "Let's count his toes. He's got ten of them. And ten fingers too!"

I couldn't stand it.

"I called ahead to explain our situation. You know this baby isn't ours, right?" I said.

"Oh, of course," she said, shaking her head up and down gravely. I thought she understood. She didn't, though. Apparently, the sight of the baby swept her away.

"He's got a perfect little heart, you can see that," she said. Sure enough, there was the powerful pulse of his beating heart. She moved the wand around, scanning for something more until his beautiful face filled the screen. "What a handsome guy! And he's got a beautiful head of hair, the little charmer."

I looked at Sean trying to get a reality check, but it was clear that he was as shaken as I was. Who could blame her? A baby is a joyful event, a cause for celebration that everyone except us could participate in, even strangers who would never see him again. Would we be strangers to this child too? No. That couldn't be, because we were both hopelessly in love with this baby.

As I drove home from the ultrasound, resentment flooded my mind. I was so distraught, and I couldn't see how I was going to rid myself of my toxic, bitter mood. I needed a break from this whole thing. I needed some time to concentrate on myself and my family, and in order to do this I was going to have to try to put Shannon out of my mind. I recognized that opening up communication with Shannon had made things harder, not easier. Shannon went on about her plans for her nursery, buying clothes for Little Man, and needing a new car in order to accommodate three car seats. I assumed that she meant no harm. She was just trying to reach out, but what she didn't realize was that her innocent messages were causing me incredible sadness and bitterness. I needed to turn away to get to a better place. The only way I could do that was to pull back on my communications with her.

The amnio was done, the 3-D ultrasound was complete, and the pregnancy was healthy. There was nothing else to do, no reason to communicate with Shannon until my next prenatal appointment in a month. I pledged to take the opportunity to focus on our own family. I would refocus my attention and energy on Drew, Ryan, and Mary Kate and on the search for a gestational carrier.

After sixteen years of marriage, Sean still surprised me from time to time, as he did when I brought up the idea of finding a surrogate. I thought we'd be arguing about it for the duration of this pregnancy, but I was wrong. All it took was three discussions and one canceled appointment before he agreed that we shouldn't waste any time and that this was the only course if we wanted to give all our embryos a chance at life. We had our lawyer Mary Smith begin a search, and I started to look at the women who had posted their biographical information on surrogacy websites. There were some afternoons when I was surfing the web for surrogates, caring for MK, and trying to manage my pregnancy symptoms and I'd just have to pause for a while to marvel at this life we were living. I wanted to get away from it. I needed some rest. I decided that as soon as we had chosen a gestational carrier I was going to get out of town. I wanted to spend some time with my mom and dad, who would be happy to take care of me, and the visit would be great for MK and the boys too.

SEAN

As I DROVE TO pick up Carolyn for the meeting with Jennifer, the woman we thought might be the right gestational carrier, I thought about the fact that a year before I didn't even know what a gestational carrier was. Now Carolyn and I were meeting a candidate to be *our* gestational carrier.

I resisted when Carolyn introduced this idea, but I know now that one reason for that reaction was that I didn't understand the process. It was more, however, than lack of understanding. With everything else going on, we didn't need another task to tackle. Slowly I embraced the idea, but only after learning more and concluding that we really had no other reasonable alternative. As I anticipated meeting Jennifer, a woman who seemed like a good candidate, I hoped the beautiful day was a good omen. The memory of the harsh and anxious winter seemed to evaporate in the seventy-degree temperatures. As we got off at the exit Carolyn's cell phone rang. It was Jennifer.

We had agreed to meet her at a spot halfway between our home and where she lived in Indiana. Carolyn picked an exit off Interstate 69 and searched the web to find a place where we could meet. She chose a Huddle House, a setting that would add another layer to the surreal experience.

"Jennifer says the Huddle House is out of business," Carolyn repeated. "She wants us to meet her at the Dairy Queen just down the road."

I nodded yes.

"Sean, what's that grimace?" Carolyn asked.

"Dairy Queen! That's a place for post–basketball game celebrations. Now we're going to use it to have one of the most important meetings of our lives."

"Nothing should surprise you about this at this point," Carolyn said. We smiled. She was right.

I pulled into the Dairy Queen parking lot and saw a neatly dressed woman with perfectly coiffed hair sitting at one of the picnic tables. Carolyn identified her instantly from the picture she'd posted on the surrogacy website. As we shook hands she stared at Carolyn, not knowing what to say about Carolyn's pregnant belly. I am sure that at that moment she was thinking: *How fast can I end this meeting? Are these people so crazy they do not realize my services are not needed?*

After exchanging handshakes and introductions, silence descended. Who was going to start?

"Well, just to get the obvious out of the way, I'm sure you noticed I am pregnant," Carolyn began. "I'm sorry we didn't tell you about this prior to now, but due to the circumstances surrounding my pregnancy, we are hesitant to put anything in writing with regards to our situation."

Jennifer looked confused and perhaps a little regretful that she had agreed to meet with us.

Carolyn explained the mistake and that after this pregnancy she wouldn't be able to carry any more children.

"Our embryos are still cryopreserved. We wanted to proceed as soon as we found the right person to help us," Carolyn continued.

"Oh, how can something like that happen? I feel so horrible for you!" Jennifer said. "Is there anything I can do to help?"

Well, yes, I wanted to say. *That is why we are here today.*

Jennifer explained her background and how she had decided to become a gestational carrier to help others.

"I've been an egg donor a few times to a fertility clinic in Indianapolis, and I'd always thought about being a carrier," Jennifer explained. "My reproductive endocrinologist recommended me to a couple in 2006, and in December 2007 I gave birth to an eight-pound baby girl. The pregnancy was textbook, and I loved giving this couple the chance to fulfill their dream. That's what made me want to do it again."

I like this woman, I thought. She seemed professional, reserved, and articulate. More than that, though, what appealed to me was her gentle nature and her genuine empathy for our predicament. She shared with us that she was a nursing student.

"Do you have any children of your own?" I asked.

"Yes, I have a daughter who is twelve," Jennifer said.

"That's the same age as our second son, Ryan," Carolyn said.

"Are you married?" I asked.

"No, I'm engaged to a man I've been with for many years," she said.

We talked about the legal aspects of surrogacy, and I was impressed by how much she knew. She wasn't put off by any of the complicated arrangements we needed her to agree to. I told her that we'd transferred our embryos out of the clinic that made the mistake and to one in Atlanta. Although the embryos were a thousand miles away, if Jennifer agreed to be our surrogate, she'd fly to Atlanta for the transfer, but she'd be monitored in Indianapolis where she lived.

"We want to be part of your pregnancy," Carolyn said. "How do you envision being involved after delivery?"

"I don't expect anything from you after the delivery except a few pictures, and maybe you can let me know how the baby is doing once a year or so. I understand that this would be your baby."

In my view, this was a perfect answer. She had found a calling in life that would help bridge things for her economically. She was involved in surrogacy for the right reasons. There was a comfortable pause after she finished speaking. Jennifer had said all the things we wanted to hear, and she seemed like a lovely person.

"Well, okay then," I said, sensing that we'd each exchanged enough information. "Let's talk on Monday after we've had the weekend to think about this and to speak with your references, including the family you worked with in 2007."

When we got back in the car, Carolyn had a huge smile on her face.

"So what did you think?" she asked me.

"I like her. A lot!"

"Me too. You know, she has such a soothing voice. That's a voice I know would be great for the baby. The baby would feel the warmth of that voice in the womb."

"I was surprised by how quickly she said she only wanted a few photos after the baby was born," I said. I liked the fact that she was in a city a good distance from Toledo. It would be awkward if we were bumping into her in the mall.

"I know, but I don't think it's going to be that way," Carolyn said. "I just can't imagine taking the baby from her at the hospital without maintaining a relationship with her. If Jennifer is our carrier, we will be connected to her forever."

"I agree!"

CAROLYN

Now that we had found a wonderful, honorable, and genuine young woman who was willing to carry our baby, I felt so happy. There were many things to arrange to make this happen, but I tackled them with joy in my heart. I called our new fertility doctor in Atlanta, who explained that there were several cumbersome FDA requirements to complete prior to getting Jennifer to a transfer. As a result, Jennifer, Sean, and I all had to fly to Atlanta to undergo numerous medical tests. Then we had to make arrangements for Jennifer to be monitored by an Indianapolis fertility clinic, as well as arrangements for Jennifer's second trip to Atlanta for the embryo transfer in early August. It was a lot of work, and it quickly became obvious to me, with some amusement, that the fastest way to get a woman pregnant with someone else's baby was to do it by accident.

Fortunately, I was able to wrap up everything that needed to be done regarding our surrogacy in time to leave it all behind, get one more ultrasound, and then retreat to my parents' home for rest and relaxation. My mom and dad live along the shores of southern Lake Michigan, and their house is something of a vacation home for us. I was ecstatic about getting away from the monotony of my day-to-day life at home, and I knew the kids would love spending the days playing on the beach, going fishing, and sailing the afternoons away on Papa's boat. Though Sean had to stay back for work and I knew I would miss seeing him daily, I really needed the escape and the extra sets of hands to help me with Mary Kate.

The surrogacy and the possibility that we might soon have a baby in our family helped me redirect my emotions. The bitterness and resentment that had consumed me for the past five months were finally giving way to hope for the future. Surely Karma would circle back around and repay us. Could Shannon be right? Could this be God's divine plan unfolding behind the scenes in a way that was meant to be? What if, through this event, my baby would be born from Jennifer and escape the dangers of a premature delivery due to the failure of my body? What if this Little Man carried to term because he didn't have a genetic link to me, sparing him the autoimmune response I had with Ryan and MK? What if Shannon's body would have failed this child? What if this child would have been doomed inside of her? Could it be that Shannon was actually right? That this was all "God's plan"?

Nope. Sometimes things just happen, and it is our job to pick up the pieces and take steps toward a better place. In order to do that I needed to stop stressing about God's plan and worry about my own, which would have to include an improved attitude.

You are turning toward hope. That is good. What next? Where do you go from here?

I had an idea, but I still wasn't sure I was strong enough to act on my new perspective just yet.

You are strong enough. You can do this. This is the right thing.

And without giving it any further thought, I grabbed my computer and frantically wrote a message to Shannon.

Hi Shannon,

> *Everything is still fine with me and the baby. I wanted to let you know that you are more than welcome to come to the ultrasound next week. As difficult as this has been for us, I think it would be okay for you to come and meet my ob/gyn and see the baby. It might take some of the mystery out of delivery day for you.*

> *Also, as for the delivery, Sean and I are gearing up for that day with our counselor. Our plan is to have you and Paul there so that as soon as the baby is ready to be taken to the nursery, you can see/meet him outside of the operating room. I seem to remember they took my daughter and my son very quickly from the room, so it would only be a few minutes from the time of delivery to the time you would be able to meet him. We'd also like some private time to say hello and good-bye to him in the operating room.*

> *As for the hospital stay, I think we can get a room arranged for you all to have with the baby in the maternity wing. This would only be overnight, or until they discharge him. It would, however, give you some privacy to bond with him as normally as this situation allows. Let me know if that is what you want, and we can start pulling the necessary strings to get this done.*

> *We have been told that it is psychologically advisable to have our*

*boys meet the baby. Just to put some concrete reason behind all of
the disruption in our lives. We would most likely do this the day of
delivery. After that, we will move on and let you all carry on with him
without disruption from us.*

    *Of course, all the above is subject to carrying to term. If anything
should happen prematurely, we will let you know immediately. You'll
be our first phone call, I promise.*

    *The appt. next week is on Monday at 1:10 pm. It is an ultra-
sound followed by a prenatal appt. with my ob. Let me know, and I
will get you directions on how to get to her office.*

                                                   Carolyn

I finished the message and surveyed my work while I wiped the
tears from my face. It was a plan, but was I really strong enough to
have Shannon at an appointment with me?

You are strong enough. This will help her.

Was it right to ask for just a moment to say "hello and good-bye"
to a child we loved so much? After all, I wanted for so much more.

*Perhaps they'll understand and honor your bond with this child. Maybe
they will have mercy on you and you'll all move forward together.*

I knew deep inside that inviting Shannon to be present at the
next appointment was the right move. Before I could give it much
more thought, I pressed Send, turned out the light, and drifted off
to sleep, satisfied in my decision to move forward, hoping it was a
sign of grace.

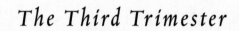

The Third Trimester

CHAPTER 14

Reaching Out

CAROLYN

THE MONTH OF JULY had given me time to think. I needed to make peace with this situation, which meant making peace with Shannon. To make this turn of mind, I relied on the feedback of my friends. My closest friends, JoAnn, Linda, Tracy, and Ann, helped me reflect on how I could escape from my pity party. In addition to those women, I also had the help of an amazing group of women from around the United States and Canada.

Originally we'd met on an IVF message board. When the pregnancy was certain, I told them first because they all had undergone IVF in order to have their families, so they had a better understanding than most of my friends of what I was going through. The news shocked them, but they rallied quickly and consistently. Most of them I had never met in person, but they became my sanity check. Many times a day we'd convene in a private Facebook group where at least one of them was always available to help me sort through my emotions and reactions. I called them my "Reliable Girls," and their support was priceless.

Suzanne, my Atlanta Reliable Girl, was the one who organized the Facebook group. She also helped us find our new fertility clinic in Atlanta and made the introduction for us so that we didn't have to cold-call and tell the story to the receptionist and everyone else who answered the phone along the way. I even stayed with her when I had to go to Atlanta for tests prior to Jennifer's transfer. The Reliable Girls counseled me through every prenatal scare and every anxiety-filled moment. Part of their value was not only their incredible ability to empathize with me but also the way they understood Shannon. Having undergone IVF themselves, they could see the challenges of both of our paths. Their advice helped me understand her, and I started to gain the perspective I needed to move forward.

After careful reflection with those closest to me, and especially the Reliable Girls, I realized I wasn't sure that I should trust my first impressions of Shannon. Although everyone agreed that some of Shannon's communication had been insensitive, they also appreciated that she too was just trying to do her best in a bad situation. I had judged her so harshly for saying how hard this was on herself, but what was happening to her was unreal too. Every day I woke up unable to believe this was my life. She must have been having those mornings too, which could explain some of her statements.

In one of Shannon's e-mails, she complained that she felt like a spectator.

Really? I'd thought. *Wait until I get to watch them take a baby out of me and give it to someone else.*

I assumed she didn't mean me any harm. Despite the counsel of some to keep Shannon at arm's length, I thought that if I did so I wouldn't be giving her a chance to understand my despair. We had met each other in a conference room surrounded by lawyers who had advised us on what to say and what not to say. If she came with me to one of my doctor's appointments, she might see how much I cared about this baby and have more empathy. Also, at Dr. Read's I routinely had an ultrasound. If Shannon came with me, she'd have a chance to see the baby alive on the screen. This might help her prepare mentally for what was going to happen in just a few months, and it might help me feel more empathy for her. Shannon agreed to my invitation eagerly.

While my local friends were so impressed that I had extended this generous invitation to Shannon, the Reliable Girls were very wary. They cited some of the e-mail exchanges I'd had with Shannon as evidence that my magnanimous gesture might not be appreciated in the way I wanted it to be. I hoped they were wrong.

The day of the appointment was warm, so I chose a pink maternity blouse and white capri pants. I thought I looked pretty good considering how I had been feeling. I was exhausted. I couldn't eat past 4:00 P.M., and I had to sleep sitting up with pillows propped around me because of acid reflux. If I turned on my side, I felt terrible. On the bright side, though, my blood pressure had remained normal. After I'd dressed and gotten MK ready, I called Dr. Read's office to alert Linda that Shannon would attend the ultrasound.

As I pulled into the doctor's office parking lot, I found Shannon waving excitedly when she recognized me. By the time I grabbed my purse, she was at my car door with a big smile on her face.

"Carolyn! I'm so happy that you invited me to come," she said.

"Hi, Shannon," I said. "I haven't got a sitter for Mary Kate, so I brought her along. Mary Kate, this is Mrs. Morell."

"Oh, what a little doll!" Shannon said. "Look at her in her cute little outfit."

I walked to the back of the car to pull out the stroller.

"Look! We have the same car seats," Shannon said. "Do you want me to get her out for you?"

"Yes, thank you," I said.

Shannon unbuckled MK and put her in the stroller for me. As we walked toward the medical building, I was worried that we had twenty minutes before the appointment. We waited on a bench outside the building. Thankfully, Shannon has the gift of gab, so I didn't have to say much at all.

I learned that Paul was an electrical engineer. Shannon's parents lived in the thumb of Michigan, close to a port that my family often visited on our sailboat. Shannon's only sister worked in a kindergarten classroom, and her brother-in-law was a principal. Her mom also worked in a school. A family of educators is a good thing in my book, as I was sure they all loved children. Eventually we got around to the subject that had brought us together.

"Well, we finally told our parents and Paul's mom, just the immediate family. That's it, though. The baby will surprise everyone else," she said. "Some people we hope never to tell. Ever. My counselor at school says that sometimes it is just better to say as little as possible.

"It's hard telling people, anyways. The few we have told always end up expressing their congratulations," Shannon continued. "It feels so weird to be congratulated on something that has been so upsetting to us. No one gets how hard this is for us. Like, we just get to show up at the hospital and bring home a baby. I wanted to be pregnant. I wanted to experience this with my girls. I have a colleague who is due a few weeks after you are. I gave her all of my maternity clothes, and I didn't anticipate how emotional it was going to be for me to give those away. I wanted to be wearing them. You know?"

"I can only imagine," I said. She and I had discussed how difficult this was for her on the phone a few months earlier, but now, listening as she brought it up again, I began to realize how much she was struggling. I was grateful that she was so comfortable opening up, but at the same time I still hesitated to tell her how often I cried or how scared I was.

She's trying, Carolyn. She's trying. You could open up.

No. I can't. I would only hurt her more.

A few minutes before my appointment, we entered the building and took our seats in Dr. Read's waiting room. Sean walked in just as we rose to go back for my ultrasound.

I lay down on the table, took a deep breath, and pulled up my shirt, revealing my pregnant belly to everyone in the room. Linda squirted the gel on my stomach, and I turned my head to watch Little Man pop up on the screen. In an instant, he was there. I glanced at Shannon, who beamed at the first live image of her son she had seen.

"Okay, little guy. Let's cooperate today and put on a good show for our guest!" Linda said.

Linda completed the basic measurements of fetal growth and amniotic fluid. She put the sensor right next to his heart, and the rhythm of his heartbeat filled the whole room. Linda then gave us a good look at the baby.

"Here are his feet. He has ten toes. This is the top of his brain. We can see all four chambers of his heart. Let me see if we can get a good look at his face."

And as if Little Man had heard her, he looked right at us, providing a perfect image of his face.

"Oh, good boy. See that? His nose, eyes, lips. We can even see his teeth in his mouth! Now, do you want a picture of his man parts?"

I started to answer, but before I could, Shannon declined. That was when I realized that Linda was talking to Shannon. The extra time looking, the commentary on what we were seeing, were all for Shannon. I turned my stare to the ceiling, beginning to feel like the third wheel, a spectator for sure.

Breathe, Carolyn. Breathe. This was the kind thing to do. Shannon needed to see this child. She needed to see that he is inside your body. This is a good thing. She will bond with her son and understand that he is bonded to you. This will help. Just breathe.

"Okay. All done," Linda said.

She handed me a towel to wipe off the ultrasound gel, and I sat up. She printed out the ultrasound pictures, and I turned to take them, but she handed them to Shannon.

We exited the room, and I went to the bathroom, shut the door, and pressed my hands to my eyes.

Get a grip, Carolyn. You invited her. It was the right thing to do. Now stop it!

I took a deep breath and went about the routines of a normal prenatal visit. I peed in a cup, stood on the scale, and sat for my blood pressure.

"Hmmmm . . . 138/80. That is the highest you've been to date."

Given the circumstances of this visit, I thought an elevated blood pressure was understandable.

Sean, Shannon, and MK were in the examining room when I entered, and MK already had her toys strewn all over the floor. Dr. Read arrived and started my routine exam. I checked out fine. Shannon remarked that my ankles looked swollen. We all studied my ankles.

"If that is as swollen as they get, you are in good shape," Dr. Read remarked.

"I'm used to being a lot more swollen by now."

"Yes, but if swelling is starting, we just want to make sure your health is protected," Shannon said. "You have this baby whenever they think it is right. We'll manage with an early delivery if we have to. That would be just fine with us."

"Well, I'm only twenty-nine weeks. A delivery right now would be a big deal, and I feel pretty good. I think we may make it with this little guy."

"I just want you to know that a premature delivery is okay with us. If we have to spend some time in the NICU, we'll deal," Shannon said.

I appreciated Shannon's sentiment. She wanted me to know that she was concerned for my health, but at the same time I don't think she understood the invasiveness of treatment in a NICU. She had taken her twins home after only three days in the hospital.

"Just to be on the safe side, I think we'll start seeing you once a week from now on," Dr. Read said.

"Sounds reasonable."

We finished the appointment and left the office.

"Thanks for coming, Shannon."

"You're welcome. It was nice to meet your doctor. Just keep me up to date on what's going on."

"Okay. Drive safely."

With that, we parted. It was all so polite, so genial, as if we were two girlfriends who had decided to share a special moment in my pregnancy. I honestly don't know how I just popped up off of the table and went on with the appointment after that confusing exchange during the ultrasound. But I did.

There were moments during this experience when I wasn't sure what I thought, and this was one of them. Yes, I had compassion for Shannon, and I could hold that feeling at the same time I experienced fear and anger and dread of what was coming. One thing was certain: I wanted to get away from all of it and try to clear my head. I wanted to rest and just concentrate on bringing this baby to term healthy and safe, nurtured by all the love I could muster. I could barely wait to get the kids packed up in the minivan so we could be on the road to my parents' Lake Michigan house.

SEAN

By the third day of coming home to an empty house, I felt melancholy. When I pulled my car into the driveway, I glanced at the basketball hoop I'd put up when we moved here. On summer evenings around this time the boys would be playing one-on-one. Most times I'd put down my work bag and shoot a few baskets with them before going into the house. Then I'd talk to Carolyn about the day while she and Mary Kate played in the backyard. Carolyn would fix dinner when I went for a run or a bike ride. I'd get home in time to spend time with the family. That was all gone for now. The silence in the house amplified my steps across the wood floor.

I changed my clothes, laced up my shoes, secured my helmet,

and threw on sunglasses. With everyone gone, I had decided to step up my training for the Sylvania Triathlon/Duathlon by increasing my workouts to one and a half to two hours. That night I planned to do a twenty-five-mile bike ride and a three-mile run. Soon I was riding past cornfields dotted with farmhouses. The corn was nearing its peak height, which meant the race was just a few weeks away. On this hot summer day, the air was thick and the corn silk tassels on top of the stalks shifted with the breeze. The aroma was sweet, and the only sound was the wind passing through my bike helmet and the occasional splat of a bug meeting its demise as it collided with the front of my helmet. In early August, when the leaves of the cornstalks started to brown, I would know that the race was upon me.

As I rode into the stiff wind, my mind went to Carolyn. The sun was just above the horizon, which meant that it was almost MK's bedtime. I pictured Carolyn with Mary Kate on her lap, reading her a bedtime story. I wanted to be with them. I started pounding the pedals harder. I pictured us like particles floating in the water of a slow-draining sink going around and around as the water slowly receded. At first, we floated at the perimeter, but we had been picking up speed all through our slow descent until we would soon be sucked into the drain. We'd dealt with so many aspects of this disaster during the previous 175 days, especially the vital decisions—the legal and medical problems, the social problems, the surrogacy—but all of that had taken place at the periphery. Time was drawing us closer and closer to the one thing we had no way to stop—the delivery and handing over of this child to the Morells. I could not wrap my mind around the delivery no matter how many times I tried to picture it.

Our lives had collided with the Morells' lives, and somehow we'd have to figure out a way to develop a friendly relationship. Carolyn and I were confused about how we should be interacting with Shannon and Paul, and our thoughts and feelings about them began to fluctuate between keeping our boundaries and letting them into our lives. Carolyn had introduced an idea to me earlier in the day during a phone call.

"I think Shannon and Paul should be in the delivery room," Carolyn said. "I don't want to deprive them of seeing their baby born."

"I understand. But it's such a private moment. Also, it's going to be a C-section, and there are many variables with your health and the baby's health."

"I think to surrender to giving this gift, I have to remove myself mentally from the scene. This is not about us or me. Maybe if they were there, I could focus on their joy, not our loss. This is our gift of life to Paul and Shannon."

"Regardless of how we do this, it is a gift. We really have to think about how this will play out in reality. The range of emotions in that room will be tremendous. I think we need that moment with you and me and the baby."

"I just don't know. I mean, it seems wrong to deny them that."

"The entire situation is wrong. Carolyn, if Paul and Shannon are in the delivery room with us, it will be like a birth and death in the same room at the same time. We may never get over that memory. I believe there needs to be separation."

"Can't we all celebrate this birth together?"

"I do not think it is possible to predict how everyone will react, including ourselves."

"I don't know. I have to think about that, Sean. You might be right."

Carolyn was so gracious to give this further consideration. I just had a gut feeling that the solution was two deliveries. The first would be with Carolyn and me, followed by a second delivery when I brought the baby to Paul and Shannon just minutes later. If that upset Paul and Shannon, I'd share with them that it was my decision, not Carolyn's.

I pedaled harder as the sun beat down and sweat soaked my shirt. This process had been beating me down mentally. For the past five months, I'd felt like I had slowly cut off blood flow to the optimistic part of my brain. When people asked how I was doing, I just said, "Okay." Not "good" or "great." "Okay" was no way to live life, and even that response was a white lie. Nothing I was experiencing seemed okay. It seemed like a living hell, actually.

After my workout, I walked through the silent house and upstairs to shower. In the mirror, I saw my weary face. These five months seemed to have aged me five years. The groom in the wedding picture in our bedroom appeared younger every time I looked at him. That's what I should have been saying when people asked me how I was doing. I could truthfully say, "I understand now how one ages."

As I settled in bed, Carolyn called. The conversations we had while she was away were always brief because they simply reminded us of our separation. Earlier that day, they had all gone to the beach, and the boys swam and played baseball while MK played with toys on a blanket. I felt my loneliness mitigated by how glad I was that Carolyn was finding some comfort around her mom and dad.

It was when I turned out the light that I missed her most of all. I thought about what life would be like if I had no family. Each night just before I fall asleep, my mind turns to prayer.

God, thank you for today. I am deeply blessed with a wonderful family and loyal friends. Please give me the courage to get up tomorrow and embrace another day and the strength to carry our cross a bit further. I need to search for more empathy for the clinic and the Morell family. Keep safe the unborn child and Carolyn and our children. Please forgive my shortcomings of the day and help those who had tragedy hit today. Please allow peace and understanding to someday enter my being.

Could I someday find peace and understanding on this journey? The silence of the empty house did not calm the turmoil within me but instead forced me to address it. I regretted all those times I had opposed Carolyn on the infertility treatments. I knew this opposition hurt her. I should have been more supportive during that part of our marriage. Family really was the most important thing in my life; I wouldn't know how to define myself in the world without it. The joking around of the boys, Mary Kate's squeals of glee—this was everything Carolyn and I wanted in the world. As I finally drifted off to sleep, I was comforted by the idea that we were trying to have another child and Jennifer was there to help us.

CHAPTER 15

Managing Two Pregnancies

CAROLYN

WHEN THE KIDS AND I returned from my parents' house in the second week of August, I found that I was suddenly managing two pregnancies: one with someone else's baby and the one we hoped for with our surrogate. I was well into my third trimester, while Jennifer was in Atlanta getting ready to have our embryos transferred into her. We'd had them shipped to our new fertility doctor in Atlanta in a cryopreservation tank. We knew so well what was happening to Jennifer that I could picture it. The incredible reality was that a transfer was taking place at the same time that I was having my weekly prenatal visit. Sean and I prayed that our embryos would survive the thaw and be of good quality. Before I entered Linda's room for my ultrasound, I checked my cell phone to make sure I hadn't missed a call from the doctor in Atlanta. He had pledged to report on the progress.

I was literally of two minds—my thoughts split right down the middle—as I watched the heartbeat of Little Man on the ultrasound screen and saw Linda take his measurements. The other half of my mind was imagining a lab technician in Atlanta carrying our embryo straw into the room where Jennifer lay on the operating table.

"You know, your placenta is still covering your cervix," Linda said, pulling me away from my imagination. "We would have hoped it would move by now. Let me get Dr. Read so she can take a look."

Linda left the room, and I looked at Sean.

"Is this bad?" he asked.

Before I could answer, Dr. Read was in the room taking a look at the ultrasound screen.

"Yup. That's a complete previa. Man. Usually placentas move off of the cervix as the baby gets bigger," she said. "This little guy is breech, and he is probably going to stay that way because there's no room for him to go head down. I'm a little concerned that we could be looking at a placenta accreta."

"What's that?" Sean asked.

Dr. Read explained that a placenta accreta is when the placenta, which usually detaches from the wall of the uterus during childbirth, remains intermingled with the uterus.

"If the placenta is too deeply attached to the uterus, we might have to perform a hysterectomy when you deliver this baby," Dr. Read said. "The danger is that giving birth to the baby would force me to cut out the placenta too, and Carolyn could hemorrhage severely, a life-threatening condition."

Sean gasped, but oddly enough, I didn't. My childbearing days were done. We all knew that. I had mourned that months before. My thoughts were on the lives we were shepherding this day. I was more worried about my embryos and Little Man.

"Could this hurt the baby?" I asked.

"Only if you start to bleed through the cervix. I am going to order an MRI to rule out the accreta. We can't do that until thirty-two weeks, so until then we will just watch and pray that we get good news from the MRI."

Dr. Read excused herself, and Sean and I exchanged befuddled expressions.

"Boy. You two just can't catch a break, and this little guy, he needs to be more cooperative," Linda said. Apparently Little Man was positioned in a way that was making the rest of the ultrasound difficult for Linda.

"Okay, little boy. You are in the wrong place," she said to my belly, and I burst out laughing.

"Linda, what do you expect? He has never been in the right place. Not from the get-go. In fact, I bet he is going to be the kid in the class who is always in the wrong place. 'Where's Little Man?' the teacher will ask when he is missing from the library. 'He went to gym, teacher!' the kids will shout back. He's going to need a map, a GPS, and a lot of directional assistance to get through life."

We were all laughing, which was a nice reprieve considering the news we had just been given and the news we were waiting to get.

As Sean and I left the office, my phone rang, and I recognized the Atlanta area code immediately.

"Carolyn, I've got good news. We thawed three of your five embryos, and you have two good-looking ones."

"Two? Does that mean one didn't survive the thaw?"

"Yes, but the two you have are looking really good. I just want to clarify. We are transferring two, right?"

"Two it is. Thanks, Dr. Straub. That is the best news I've had all day."

I hung up, looked at Sean, and smiled. Two embryos survived the thaw, and now I had two more unborn lives to pray for. I felt incredibly lucky.

After the transfer, the clinic e-mailed me an image of the embryos. When I got the images, I studied them.

I rummaged through my files and found the pictures of Mary Kate's embryo. They didn't look anything alike.

MK was a five-day-old embryo. These were two-day embryos, which were smaller and had far fewer cells. MK had over one hundred cells at the time of transfer. These embryos only had two cells. I couldn't compare them. What about Little Man's embryo picture?

I opened Sean's CF binder and right away I found the picture of the embryos transferred into me in February, thanks to my husband's handy organizational system. I removed the picture from the plastic sleeve and stared at it. I hadn't seen it since the embryo transfer, when I held it and prayed for my potential babies. I took note of the label attached to the bottom that had all of our personal information on it, including my date of birth, which I recognized—again—as wrong. And once again, I also wondered about what could have been, what should have been.

The embryos kind of looked the same, I realized, although my embryos had less fragmentation than Little Man's. Because he'd been a five-day-old embryo, Little Man had ten to twelve cells at the time of the transfer. *Well, if he can come out of a poor-grade embryo,* I thought, *surely one of these could turn into a baby for our family.*

I printed the picture, cut it out so that it was the size of an index card, labeled it "Carolyn and Sean Savage's Embryos," and hung it on the bulletin board next to my computer. They represented hope. Human potential. I was glad they were in Jennifer and thanked God for bringing her into our lives. She was truly an angel to us, and I would never, ever forget what she was doing for our family.

Two weeks later, the nurse called to tell me that Jennifer's pregnancy hormones—her beta HCG—measured 90. Definitely pregnant! As I heard the words come out of the nurse's mouth, it was as if my world righted itself. I had never been so thankful for a phone call in my entire life. Maybe this was the way it was supposed to be. A baby was coming to our family.

Two days later, Jennifer underwent another blood test to make sure her pregnancy hormones were still rising. This time the nurse's tone was guarded. "The HCG level is going up, but not as quickly as we would like to see. We are going to test her again on Friday."

The blood work was acceptable, though, so there was still hope.

Two days later, the nurse's tone was cautionary. The HCG was still going up, but again, not at the rate they would have liked to see.

"The doctor will test her again on Monday."

It was a long wait that weekend, but like a trooper, Jennifer went in for a fourth blood draw, and we both waited anxiously that Monday afternoon. The call came to my cell.

It's going to be okay. Have faith.

"Carolyn, we have terrific news for you. The beta level was 700 today. That is right on schedule. Congratulations!"

I thanked her for calling and hung up to call Sean.

"Hey. All is perfect. Her levels are right where they are supposed to be!"

"What a relief!" was all he could manage.

"They are going to check it again next Monday, and then she'll have an ultrasound on September 3, to check for a heartbeat."

I rubbed my belly, talking to Little Man. "You are going to have a buddy, Little Man! Thanks for pulling some strings for us!"

As my pregnancy progressed, Dr. Read thought it would be advisable to involve a perinatologist, a high-risk obstetrician, in my care. The new doctor suggested that I have appointments twice a week to catch even the most subtle changes immediately. Sean and I were happy with the plan, even though it required a lot of me. My mom had moved in with us for the rest of the pregnancy, no matter how long or short it was going to be. Having her around freed me up to rest and to attend my appointments without dragging Mary Kate around. The perinatologist said he'd probably schedule my C-section at thirty-seven weeks.

Thirty-seven weeks? I couldn't imagine that I would get that far.

The following Monday I got another call from the nurse in Atlanta. "Well, the news is not good. Jennifer's HCG is only 3,500. We would have expected it to be over 5,000 by now. The ultrasound is on Thursday. Just know, we are all pulling for you."

I hung up the phone feeling like I had been sucker-punched. How could this be God's plan? I ran the test results by Dr. Read at my appointment later that day, and she expressed concern. On the bright side, Little Man passed his nonstress test with flying colors, and he looked great in the ultrasound. All we could do with regard to our baby was pray and wait until Thursday.

Jennifer's appointment on September 3 was at 2:00 P.M. I had a 1:45 appointment with the perinatologist. I was so nervous waiting for the results of Jennifer's ultrasound that I couldn't concentrate on anything else, and I was surprised to notice that my anxiety was not reflected in my blood pressure reading.

"We are going to start with the nonstress test!" I lay back on the table while the nurse positioned the belts across my rather large pregnant belly. "You have to stay hooked up for at least twenty minutes," she explained. "So, lie back, relax, and try not to talk."

I pressed my phone to my chest, closed my eyes, and prayed. *Please, God. Please let my baby live. Please let my baby live.*

A few minutes passed as I listened to Little Man's heart beat strongly on the monitor and pondered the ridiculousness of this situation. I wondered if, in the history of mankind, a woman had ever been hooked up to a fetal monitor while waiting for a call from another woman about her own baby's heartbeat? I continued to pray for both heartbeats, and when the phone rang, both Little Man and I jumped.

"Carolyn? Great news. We have one healthy heartbeat!"

Jennifer gave me more details, but I wasn't paying attention. Joy and relief had overtaken my heart. Her transfer had resulted in one baby who had a robust heartbeat, and Little Man's was strong too. What more could a mother ask for?

I left that appointment with a clean bill of health from the doctor and an unburdened heart. Now I had two babies growing. How blessed was I?

SEAN

As the door to the office closed behind us and we entered the hall-way, we both were upbeat. I reached for Carolyn's hand as we went down the hall and squeezed it as a sign that we were going to get through this. Carolyn walked with conviction, and I saw a positive look on her face for the first time since the beginning of the ordeal. Together, we were willing ourselves to higher ground.

I got back into my car very relieved for this ray of hope for our family and its future. Then I was quickly sucked back into the present. I was thumbing through e-mails that I had previously received and came to the one that was making my heart skip a beat: a follow-up e-mail from George Tanber, a Pulitzer Prize–winning journalist. George had originally contacted us in July when he had learned about our situation and asked if he could write about us. We declined, and now, as all good journalists do, he was making a second request. I knew word of our pregnancy was spreading. Just a few days ago a client of mine, someone who didn't even live in the area, tearfully told me that she was sorry for what she'd heard was happening to Carolyn and me.

I knew we were lucky that George had been so respectful of our privacy, but realized that the next reporter might not be as gracious. His follow-up request was our wake-up call. We had a choice to make: play defense and react to calls as they came and risk having our story told inaccurately by a third-rate tabloid, or go on offense and tell our story ourselves. We chose offense.

Carolyn and I first consulted with local public relation experts, Mike Hart and Matt Schroder, who told us that it wasn't a question of whether or not our story would be in the press, but when. They believed that it might even become an international story. I asked them to recommend an attorney who specialized in media relations, and they put us in touch with an attorney in New York, who convinced us that we needed to hire a New York public relations firm. The New York PR firm advised us to get out in front of the story so that no one could try to tell it for us. We took their advice.

Our charge to these advisers was simple. We wanted to speak with no one but the most professional journalists, people who would have compassion for our situation. The New York firm took over those arrangements for us, and we were very pleased to have that worry off our backs.

That night Carolyn was still awake when I came up to bed.

"Aren't you excited that we have a child coming?" she asked.

"I am very excited, honey, but there's still anxiety," I said. "What if the pregnancy fails? Are we setting ourselves up for a small lift and a big fall?"

For me, it was tough to imagine that there would be something positive happening with another child down the road. Suddenly good news was foreign to us. On the other hand, the one thought that did cross my mind was that with all of the difficulty we had faced that year, I could not imagine anything else going wrong.

I was nearly asleep when Carolyn said, "Sean, I ordered the baby a gift today."

"What kind of a gift?" I asked.

"I ordered him a cashmere receiving blanket. It's light blue with a satin edge, and I wrote a message to have embroidered on each side. I must have written those four lines at least a hundred times before I got it just right," Carolyn continued. "It starts, 'Little Man, Although our time together was brief.' I want him to know that, even though he isn't our genetic son and we won't get to raise him, the time that we had with him bonded him to us and us to him.

"The next line is 'Know your life is a gift, your birth a blessing,'" she continued. "He has to know that his life, his existence, was never a burden to us.

"'And know our love flies to you on angels' wings,'" she said. I saw there were tears in her eyes. "I want him to know that he will never leave our thoughts, and even though we can't tell him that he is adored, we will love him in our hearts and send our love to him in our prayers.

"Then it says, 'God Speed . . . Sweet Dreams . . . We'll love you forever!'" Carolyn concluded. "Most of all, I want him to have the blessings of God. I want him to close his eyes at the end of every day knowing he is treasured by a mommy and a daddy far, far away while he sweetly drifts off to sleep. He needs to know our love for him will be eternal."

A good-bye present had been ordered. Clearly the time was starting to draw nearer, and I was very aware that I was not ready.

"I hope it will be his favorite blanket," she said. "That he'll take it everywhere. But even if he doesn't, at least when he looks at it when he's older he'll know we loved him. If that blanket could have had eight sides, I would have filled every one of them with messages that I am desperate for him to know, but there was only so much a seamstress could fit in the space allowed."

"Carolyn, that is a beautiful gift, and the message is perfect," I said as tears streamed down my face. I hugged her, and we held on to each other as we drifted off to sleep.

CHAPTER 16

Facing Fear

CAROLYN

WHEN LITTLE MAN and I got to thirty-five weeks, I was shocked that I had made it that far. My original goal had been thirty-two weeks, so when we got to September, I was chalking up bonus time. If my body helped him escape the tortures of the NICU, it would be a huge achievement for me, something I wasn't able to do for MK and Ryan. I so much wanted to do that for this child. I started monitoring myself carefully—though "obsessively" might be another word for how I was behaving. Every morning I took my blood pressure before I got out of bed, the first of dozens of readings throughout the day. I wouldn't let thirty minutes go by without checking on the baby and my pregnancy. I even brought my blood pressure cuff with me in the car.

The good news was that the MRI showed that my placenta was fine, not an accreta. That same scan gave us other disturbing news, though.

"See that image there?" said the midwife who was on staff at my perinatologist's office, pointing at the screen. "Your baby's cord is wrapped around his neck four times."

I panicked when I saw the coils of cord around his neck, like rings. I knew that cord wraps were common, but I also had three friends who tragically had delivered full-term babies who were still-born because of cord accidents.

"What can I do?" I asked, frantic. "Is there any way to help him?"

"It is quite common. We probably wouldn't even know the extent of the cord wraps if it wasn't for the MRI," the midwife advised me. "The only thing you can do is keep doing your kick counts. If you notice that his activity level is dropping, call us immediately."

Kick counts. What a joke. I never understood the point of counting the kicks the baby made inside the womb. By the time the baby stopped moving, wouldn't he already be gone? What the heck was I supposed to do? Lie still all day and tally his movements? And to make matters worse, Little Man was something of an acrobat. I didn't know if it was because he couldn't settle into a head-down position or because he was going to be an Olympic gymnast. His flipping and kicking concerned me once I knew about the cord around his neck. Could all his antics pull the cord so tight that he cut off blood flow?

I decided not to share this very stressful piece of information with the Morells. The midwife was probably right that this was not going to harm him. Despite my friends' tragic outcomes, most babies seem to have the cord around their neck at some point, so I didn't feel that I had to worry Paul and Shannon.

This heightened my focus on Little Man, though. Of course, he was very rarely out of my thoughts, but now I made a mental note of his every move. When he flipped, I'd look at my watch. If he kicked, I looked at my watch. I checked my watch on the half-hour, and if I hadn't felt him, I'd drink cold water. I felt bad sending the icy fluid into his warm and cozy environment, but it always worked. He hated it! As soon as the cold water hit, he'd start kicking.

"Sorry, Little Man. I just need to know you are okay."

On September 17, I was back at my perinatologist for another appointment. They escorted me back right away for my nonstress test. The nurse, one I'd never met before, positioned the heart rate monitors on my right lower abdomen.

"You know, we always attach those on my upper left side. My baby is breech and seems to prefer to be over here," I said, pointing to the place where they usually got a good reading on Little Man.

"Oh, he's so big now, we can pretty much attach these any-where."

She finished attaching the nodes and left me alone. I noticed that Little Man was not moving a lot at the moment. I reached for my purse to pull out my water, but then I realized that I didn't have my water bottle. The nurse came in and looked at the fetal monitoring strip.

"He's not cooperating very well. We seem to keep losing his heartbeat."

"Maybe we can move the nodes to the other side?"

"Let's give him some more time," she said as she left the room.

I was growing anxious, even though I knew he was fine. I tried moving the nodes myself, but that didn't help. The nurse returned and suggested that we stimulate him. I assumed she was going to get me some ice water, as that is what the nurses at Dr. Read's office did to stimulate him. When the nurse returned, she had a contraption that looked something like a Taser.

"What is that?"

"We use this to stim the babies when they're not cooperating."

What? Before I could ask any more questions, she pressed the stun gun thing against my belly, and pushed a button. The sound that screamed out from this little machine was one of the most of-fensive sounds I had ever heard. Little Man jumped in my womb and then began a series of movements that indicated to me that he had been scared to death and was probably wailing inside of my body.

"What the hell was that?"

"Oh, don't worry. It doesn't hurt the baby. Just scares them a bit so we can see the heart rate go up."

Scare him? Why on earth would you want to scare a little baby when a dunk in cold water would have the same effect? I didn't like this approach at all, and neither did Little Man. His heart rate definitely went up, and he was thrashing around like a fish caught in a net.

"It worked," the nurse said happily. "His heart rate is definitely up. Now we just need to see it come down."

Which proved to be a problem. This nurse had just scared the hell out of this child, and I was beyond angry. As we hit the half-hour mark and his heart rate had not decelerated, we decided to call it quits and just do the ultrasound.

I lay on the table, still shaken by the thought of the baby being Tasered by the nurse, when the ultrasound technician, whom I had never met before, entered the room. She asked me what my amniotic fluid had been measuring with Linda a few days prior.

"Linda said it was twelve. It was really good."

"Have you been drinking a lot? Have you felt any leakage?"

"I've been guzzling ice water, and there hasn't been any leakage. Why?"

"Just lie still," she said. "I'm going to get the doctor."

My anxiety started to spike. By the time she returned with the doctor, I was shaking.

"Let's take a look," he said, studying the pockets of amniotic fluid in my uterus.

This can't be happening. My blood pressure is acceptable. Little Man is moving. I listen to his heartbeat on my monitor twenty times a day. Please, God . . . no problems now. I'm not ready. I'm not ready.

"Carolyn, it appears your amniotic fluid has dropped from a twelve to a seven in only three days. Seven is on the low side of the normal range. This, combined with the fact that we had a difficult time tracing your baby during the nonstress test, is cause for concern," the doctor said. "I am going to admit you."

I started to panic. I wasn't ready for this child to be born. I wasn't ready to say good-bye.

"But, are you sure? I mean, the nodes were constantly falling off, and then the nurse stunned him with that gun thingy, and he practically tried to crawl out of my uterus he was so scared. He just wouldn't hold still. Can't we just try again?"

"It really would be better to just admit you to labor and delivery, hook you up to their machinery, and get a better look at what is going on."

They must have sensed that I was planning an escape, because they escorted me, like a criminal, to the seventh floor of Mercy St. Vincent Medical Center and admitted me to the maternity ward, advising me that delivery might take place later that night.

When I entered my room, the nurse handed me a hospital gown and said I couldn't have anything else to eat or drink. This was not good news because I was starving. While she promptly hooked me up to the fetal monitors, another nurse took my vitals, and a third nurse entered the room, carrying a clipboard and a pen.

"Hi! I'm going to ask you the questions that we ask all who are about to deliver. Okay?"

I nodded yes. I remembered fifteen years ago, almost to the exact day, when I entered the very same hospital after going into labor with Drew. I hadn't gone through this intake process since then, because Ryan's and MK's deliveries were emergencies. When there is an emergency, they save these questions for later.

The nurse started with the basics: name, address, religious affiliation. I quickly spit out my answers, knowing in my heart that this baby was not coming today. The monitors were showing that Little Man was doing just fine. No need to worry. While I was giving the nurse my basic information, I wondered if these two knew about our situation. I decided that since I was certain that the delivery was not happening immediately, I wasn't going to spill the beans about this whole mess and get all emotional.

"Do any genetic members of your baby have diabetes, blood-clotting disorders, or heart eurythmias?"

I don't know.

"No."

"Are you going to breast-feed or bottle-feed?"

I think he's being bottle-fed? Not sure.

"Bottle-feed."

"Who will be his pediatrician?"

I don't know that either.

"Kiron Torsekar." The name of our pediatrician.

"Will you have him circumcised?"

God, I hope so.

"Uh . . . I think so?"

"What is the name you have chosen for your son?"

Then it hit me. *I don't know his name. How could I not know his name?*

"Not sure yet."

He's not coming today. You can do this.

"Okay, last question. Is there anything else you think we need to know about this pregnancy?"

I pressed my hands to my face in an attempt to push back my tears, but I fell into sobs in a matter of seconds.

"Well, you see, this baby isn't mine. I got pregnant with the wrong baby as a result of a botched IVF. My fertility doctor put the wrong embryos in me, and now I'm pregnant with someone else's baby."

I could hardly get the words out. The nurses exchanged glances.

Finally one of them asked, "Are you giving him up for adoption?"

This question flabbergasted me. "Hell no. We want him, but he's not ours. His genetic parents want him. We know who they are. They know who we are. They are taking him away as soon as he is delivered."

By this time I was so hysterical that my nose had turned into a faucet and my blood pressure soared to its highest reading yet.

"I tried not to say anything about this to you. But the truth is, I don't know the answers to any of the questions you asked. I'm not ready for this. I can't have this baby today. I'm not ready to let him go."

The nurse doing my vitals was sympathetically rubbing my arm and asked me to roll over on my left side to lower my blood pressure. I did as she asked and wiped my face with a tissue and looked over toward the nurse asking me the questions, who was sitting on the couch with her head in her hands, quietly crying.

I looked at the other nurse, who was trying to maintain her composure, but miserably failing. Within another minute, we were all crying and no one could talk.

A few minutes had passed when one of them said, "Well, we are a sorry bunch."

The comment enabled us to laugh halfheartedly.

"I am so sorry," said the nurse who was asking the questions. "I didn't know that could happen. You see, I've done three IVFs and a number of frozen embryo transfers to try to have a family."

"Do you have any children?" I asked.

"Yes, but we never had one of our own. We finally gave up and adopted."

"Oh. That's wonderful. Congratulations. How old is your child?" I asked as I wiped my tears away.

"We have a two-year-old son. He is the love of our lives. Do you understand what a tremendous gift you are giving to this other family?"

"Yes. We get it. We know what is right, even though it is breaking our hearts."

"Well, I get it too. What you are doing is amazing. I hope this other family has been kind to you. Do they understand what you've done for them?"

That was another question that I didn't have an answer for.

"I don't know. I hope so. Time will tell."

We finished our cry fest just as Sean walked in with my bag. I explained that I had had a bit of a meltdown, but in spite of my hysterics, the baby looked great on the fetal monitors. We had pretty much been told that we wouldn't be delivering that night but had to wait for Dr. Read to come to the hospital, lay eyes on me, and give them permission to discharge me.

When she arrived, it was well after midnight, and we were exhausted.

"I'm so sorry I made you wait. I had a delivery across town and knew I couldn't be here right away, but needed to see you for myself to make sure you were okay."

"No worries. This was a good dry run. I never even called the Morells. I knew he wasn't coming tonight. It did make me realize that I needed to get more prepared for this. I wasn't mentally ready."

"Well, everything considered, I think you need to get ready. If your blood pressure is elevated at any time from now forward, that would be enough to call for the C-section considering the drop you've had in your fluid."

"I figured that. You know, I think I need one more week. Thirty-six weeks would be a great accomplishment for me. I think September 24 or 25 sounds like a good day to be born. By then I will have cleared all of my goals. I will have made it to term, gotten past Drew's fifteenth birthday, and hopefully gotten ready to say good-bye."

Dr. Read told me she understood how important it was for me to give the baby that week to grow, but she said I had to recognize that, considering all the other factors, we could expect a delivery any day.

We drove home from the hospital that night, exhausted and relieved. My Little Man was still with me. I knew I needed to drink up these last few days with him.

CHAPTER 17

The Best Way Out Is Through

CAROLYN

MY UNEXPECTED ADMISSION TO the hospital forced us to face the fact that the baby could be arriving any day. There were many ways in which we were very well prepared. Sean had handled the logistics on all fronts in a way that left nothing to chance, but emotionally I felt as though perhaps there was no way for us to prepare for this loss.

Although Little Man had only been with us for a short time, he meant so much to us. He had profoundly affected our lives and our family, and I could not predict how he would change our future. After he left us, surely we would grieve, but what would that grief feel like?

I'd known mothers who had a baby stillborn, and I'd seen them grieve the emptiness that created. The baby who dies becomes the container for all the unfulfilled potential in life. Some mothers mourn by idealizing that child, conjecturing what kind of person that baby would have become and how much joy the family would have had as the child grew. Though we thought we were facing that kind of loss, we knew that the baby would live on beyond that moment, but nurtured by other parents. How do you mourn the loss of someone who still lives? And who goes on to give joy to another family?

People sometimes compared our situation to putting a baby up for adoption, yet that was so off the mark from what we felt. Women who give their babies up for adoption have very specific reasons for doing so. Of course their feeling of loss is great, and many of those women grieve over the fact that they couldn't afford or accommodate the new life they created. But we had the means and the space in our hearts and in our home to keep this child.

As the baby spun and twirled and kicked inside my womb, I had moments of pure pride for having managed to bring him this far. I was the woman who was about to launch this powerful Little Man into the world. That ecstatic moment when I'd hear his first cry, see him take his first breath, would be a victory for Sean and me. But what would the moments after that be like? When they cut the cord that connected him to me, he would never be mine again legally, physically, or emotionally. Yet as far as I was concerned, he would always be our baby. I knew Sean felt the same way. What kind of empty space would his departure leave behind? Every time I thought about it, I had to turn my mind away. I could feel myself falling into that loss, and there was no way out, no place for my hands to grab on to that would allow me a chance to pull myself back out.

One morning I was about to leave for our appointment with Kevin when I realized that I hadn't given myself my morning shot of blood thinners for my blood-clotting disorder. I'd recently had to switch to twice-a-day shots of Heparin because the perinatologist said Heparin was safer in the third trimester.

At first giving myself shots had been fine, if a little stomach-turning. But when I had to do it twice a day, I had a hard time finding a place to insert the needle. The injections toughened my skin. My stomach and thighs were covered with welts and bruises that made the injections become more and more painful. Just before MK was about to wake up, I sat in the bathroom, syringe in hand, trying to find a bruise-free place on my leg, when I dropped the syringe and it plunged into my foot.

The pain was unimaginable, as if someone had just stabbed me in the ankle. After I pulled it out, I threw it at the wall and burst into tears. In that moment, I had nothing left. How could I endure all of this and not get a baby? After a few minutes, and many tears, I quieted down. I was stronger than this. I had proven it already, and we were almost done. I took a deep breath, loaded a new syringe, eventually found a place to take the shot, and switched to the task at hand: packing up MK for our final prenatal visit with Kevin Anderson.

I felt depleted and gloomy as I pulled into the church parking lot for our appointment with Kevin. I was weary physically and emotionally. On the one hand, I was so happy that Little Man and I had made it this far, and there was so much of me that wanted the pregnancy to be over. Then there was another part of me that didn't want the pregnancy to be over. I wanted to stay connected to my Little Man. I was so weary of all of it and of having to be counseled. There had been sessions when we were feisty and combative, and others when we sobbed. We'd even had our share of laughter at the absurdity of some of what was going on. This session felt somber. We almost didn't know where or how to begin.

"I'm so scared," I said. "I don't know how I'm going to handle everything that happens to me after the baby is gone. My body will be a wreck, and my hormones will be raging with maternal instincts that are too powerful to turn off."

"Night after night the same vision comes to me," Sean said. "A series of quick scenes flash in my head: Carolyn being carted to surgery, me with her in the delivery room, and then a fog comes with me not being able to picture anything. Then I'm shutting the door behind the room the Morells are in with the baby boy. A wave of anger flashes through me, and I become disoriented. I walk down a hallway with a storm blowing up inside me. With all of my force, I shove my fist as fast as possible into the wall. As my fist hits the wall, I scream, 'No! No!' I see a dent as I put my back on the wall and slide down it. When I hit the floor, I take my knees to my chest and place my hands in my face and cry."

Kevin looked at the floor, folded his hands, and thought in silence.

"Who would blame me? How am I supposed to give a baby away? How is anyone supposed to give a baby away they want to raise? I've kept all of this bottled up the whole time Carolyn has been pregnant because there were more important things for me to manage than these emotions. The only question that remained was whether my fist would punch a hole through the wall or if I would simply make a dent. Yet I know a lot of people will think we will simply be relieved this is over. We should just get on with our lives as though nothing ever happened. I don't know how we'll ever be able to do that."

"'The best way out is through.' Are you familiar with that Robert Frost poem?" Kevin asked.

"No," said Sean quickly. Once again, Sean looked cranky that Kevin was citing a passage from spirituality or literature that he didn't know. He looked at me, the language arts teacher, as if I ought to know the line, but I hadn't a clue.

"It is a line from the poem 'Servant to Servants,'" Kevin said. "It's about a woman who shoulders a big burden of work.

> By good rights I ought not to have so much
> Put on me, but there seems no other way.
> Len says one steady pull more ought to do it
> He says the best way out is always through

We looked at him for a few seconds, waiting for him to explain to us what he meant.

"When I consider the options that have been available to you, those lines seem to fit your situation," he said. "You see, you could have made the choice to terminate, because it would have been easier. You didn't because that would have been wrong. You could have made the choice not to reach out to the Morells, because it would have been easier to protect yourselves from the people who could hurt you the most. You didn't because that would have been unkind. You could have refused to develop an attachment to this child because it would have lessened the blow of his departure. You couldn't because you love him. Now you are faced with the unknown. What lies ahead? Your surrogate could miscarry. The Morells could take the baby, never allowing you to see him again, and your actions could be exploited by others for personal gain. All of that could go wrong, but my guess is that you'll get through those possible disasters."

"Well, of course we'll survive them," I said. "We'll still be alive, and we'll still have our family and our work. But through? What do you mean by through?"

"You have to face it, all of it, all the emotions," he said. "When people tell you that you should be feeling a certain way or behaving in the way they would, that's not where your focus should be. Whatever you are feeling, if it's sorrow or grief or that you want to punch your fist through the wall, all of that is completely justifiable. Don't restrict the way you feel to fit someone else's agenda, someone else's idea of conduct. The best way out is through these emotions. Fully experience them, fully feel everything you feel. Only if you do that will you be able to get to the other side of this traumatic experience. The best way out *is* through. You will get there, and in the end you'll be all right."

We knew Kevin was right. We'd been fighting and kicking every day as new developments occurred. We had yet to surrender to what was coming. We didn't need to fight it. We would get out, some day, but first we had to go through.

Would we ever get past "the through"? Time would tell. I was sure scared of what was coming with the delivery and prayed again that I would have the strength to get through it.

SEAN

I AM A LONG-DISTANCE runner. At the end of the race, getting through means keeping focused and sticking to the plan I made, fighting through the pain and the urges to give up. We needed to find the willpower to get through to the end, wherever it might be. When I focused on the goal and all we needed to do to get through, I was less likely to fall into despair. The key element I needed for me to "get through" handing the baby boy over to the Morells was to focus on the gift. If I could keep the idea that this was a gift and place it alongside the pain, I believed I could honor this child and the Morells while still acknowledging a profound personal loss. There was dignity in this approach, but it would take every ounce of energy in that moment for me to achieve this balance.

As I wrapped my mind around holding these two ideas simultaneously, I knew Carolyn and I were moving forward, despite everything, and closer to being able to let go. As we approached the end of the pregnancy, we had other signs our family was moving forward. September 22 was Drew's fifteenth birthday.

There had been precious few celebrations in the last few months as we tried to keep a low profile around town. But we had allowed the world back into our lives when we finally gave interviews to the many media sources that were interested. We were on the front page of the local paper, on numerous national and international broadcasts, and the story had gone viral on the Internet. The night before Drew's birthday had been a crazy scene in our home. While we were completing an interview with a pair of journalists on our patio, another waited on our driveway, a network was setting up cameras for a live national interview in our living room, and an international camera crew was on the front lawn.

Even though the media world was swirling around our situation that week, on September 21 we would give our son the best possible birthday. Carolyn's mother was in town, so both grandmas could join us too.

Drew selected the restaurant, and as we sat at the table and shared "Drew stories" there were eyes on us. But no one bothered us as we celebrated. After dinner we all came home for cake, and in keeping with Savage tradition, Drew sat at the kitchen table behind the cake to have his picture taken holding up the number of fingers for his age. Of course, at age fifteen he needed some help. I crouched behind him, and as he held up his ten fingers I held up five over his head, totaling fifteen. Our son was fifteen. Hard to believe.

Carolyn and I made our way to bed at about 9:30 P.M. We were exhausted, and we knew that the next morning we would be doing another live national interview for a morning show. Carolyn was in the bathroom, and I was pulling clothes out for the next day when she screamed and came flying out from the bathroom.

"I think my water broke!"

"We need to get to the hospital," I said.

"Sean, grab the phone. I need to call Dr. Read."

I ran to get the phone and brought it to her. I paced the floor quickly, doing nothing close to productive. Then I grabbed the bag she had packed for the hospital and positioned it next to our bedroom door about five feet from its previous spot, like that was really helpful.

Dr. Read told us to get to the hospital. This was the real deal.

Within minutes, Carolyn and I were in the car. As we made the drive, it hit me.

"Carolyn, we cannot have the baby on Drew's birthday. This is not fair to Drew or fair to us. We can't have this happen on the same day that has one of our best memories. This would be cruel."

"I know."

My hands clenched the steering wheel so hard that I thought I might break it off of the car. I hated that we couldn't control this. If Carolyn's water had broken, they had to deliver the baby.

Carolyn called the Morells to let them know that they needed to get down to Toledo. The maternity ward was ready for us when we arrived. They hooked Carolyn to the baby monitor while we waited for Dr. Read. The sound of the baby's beating heart filled the room while I sat on the couch next to Carolyn's hospital bed. It was 10:00 P.M.

"Oh man, Carolyn," I realized. "We're scheduled to do an interview with a TV crew tomorrow morning at the house."

"Call the producer to cancel. I think they will understand."

I called and discovered that the crew was already on its way from Chicago. They agreed to turn the truck around. I apologized.

As we waited, my mind went to Drew. What would he feel like sharing a birthday with a brother he would never know? Suddenly I was really pissed at God. After everything we had gone through, and would go through in the future, how could He possibly connect this date to the delivery? We had tried to be good and faithful servants and taken the hard but noble path. I did not ask to be spared the experience—just to be spared this experience on this day.

When Dr. Read walked in the room, I stood and said in complete seriousness, "You have to wait one hour and forty-seven minutes to deliver this baby."

"Sean, I'm sorry. I don't think that's possible. If the baby is in distress, we'll have to move quickly."

She asked Carolyn a series of questions and said she was going to order a few tests.

A short while later, after reviewing the test results, she returned.

"You will not be having the baby tonight," Dr. Read said. "The tests show that your water didn't break and that the baby is still doing well."

I was so relieved and thanked God for the reprieve. That night I was pleased to have to walk the "amateur walk of shame" that happens when you arrive at the hospital pregnant and leave the hospital the same night still pregnant. I immediately called Shannon to tell her to turn around. "The baby will not be born tonight," I said and apologized for the inconvenience. Then I called the TV network, and they turned their truck back around again.

The media was certainly a presence in our lives now, and we were trying to handle it as best we could. On September 24, two days after the false alarm, I arrived at my office about 6:15 in the morning to get work done prior to meeting Carolyn at our local publicist's office for a series of local and brief television interviews. Just as I did every morning, I glanced at our local paper, *The Blade,* and I saw the front-page headline with a picture of us. But then I saw another headline, and I clutched the paper as I saw what I had hoped would never surface. The article was about the Catholic Church and the issue of IVF: "In Vitro Fertilization Poses Ethical, Religious Dilemmas." "Oh, here we go," I said out loud as I quickly read the article line by line.

The paper had obtained a statement from the Diocese of Toledo calling IVF "morally unacceptable." My interpretation of that statement was: what Sean and Carolyn Savage did in undergoing IVF was "morally unacceptable." The statement went on to explain the Church's position: in vitro fertilization is morally unacceptable because it replaces rather than assists the marital act, the diocese said.

One part of the statement especially infuriated me:

Human life is something precious. A new human being who comes into existence at the moment of conception, is meant to enter into this world within the context of committed marital love, a love which finds its fullest expression in the intimacy of the marital act. Any technique that severs the creation of a new human life from this most intimate context is not morally acceptable and ought never to be done.

I felt that this statement was laced with arrogance, and it put a knife right into our backs at a very vulnerable moment in our life. I imagined my response: *Dear Diocese, Carolyn and I have had a committed marital love for seventeen years. We wanted to have a family with a number of children that we could raise to be faith-filled, productive, and good members of society. We needed help having those children. That help we believe came from God through science. Our daughter born in March 2008, is beautiful and adored and an IVF baby. When Carolyn and I first looked into her eyes the day she was born, we saw God's creation!*

I called Carolyn immediately, and we talked about the article. We agreed that what hurt the most was what was missing from the statement. We chose life on February 16, 2009. In deciding as we did, we upheld the Church's teachings on the beauty and sanctity of human life. Why was that missing from the statement? We are members of the Church, and hurting members at that. Yet our very own church was not there to support us in our time of greatest need. Is this how Jesus would have handled us? I don't think so.

As I traveled to the PR firm for the interviews, the hurtful articles would not leave my mind. The words cut through me like a sharp knife. Over the years, Carolyn and I took to heart our stewardship responsibilities to the Church by giving our time, energy, and resources. Ministering to the youth through coaching sports, raising funds for parish expansion, and giving to worthy church causes was embedded in my being. Carolyn had dedicated much of her career to being a teacher and then a principal in Catholic schools. Now, in a public forum, we were being called out by the hierarchy of the Catholic Church to account for our "morally unacceptable" behavior. It really hurt and we felt abandoned.

Despite feeling abandoned by our church, we understood those who judged us were very distant from Carolyn and me, high up in the Church hierarchy. At St. Joe's, we received council and prayers from our clergy and support from our fellow parishioners. The people of St. Joe's were there for us. We knew we would remain members of the Church with its flaws because the Catholic Church did so much good locally and throughout the world. As word spread about our situation to places across the globe, prayers and support poured in. These warmed our hearts and touched our souls. Carolyn and I were humbled that people responded in such a loving manner. As I arrived at the PR firm for the interviews I saw Carolyn waiting for me near the front door of the building, and it hit me that this may be the last day I ever see my wife pregnant.

CHAPTER 18

Reaching Toward Joy

CAROLYN

THE BABY WOULD BE born any day, and I focused on one concern: I wanted to be fully present for every moment and have that brief period as a kind of movie that I could play again and again whenever I felt like it. I knew that our moments in the delivery room might be our only time together, and I wanted that movie to be a joyful one, one with a happy ending. We were going to take photographs of this event for us and for him. I didn't want to be a wreck. I wanted those pictures to show us as we truly felt. Despite everything that had happened, his presence on earth was a gift. When he was older and he had a chance to look at the faces of the people who brought him into this world, I hoped he would see that we were honored to give him life and that we loved him with all our hearts.

Sean's preparations, all the ways in which he had planned so carefully for the moment of the birth, were about to come to a close. On the morning of September 24, our local public relations firm had arranged for us to speak to the local television stations. I was going to meet Sean at the public relations office that morning at 8:00, and we would be done by 9:30 A.M. All of them would have had their little piece of this story, and then, we hoped, they would leave us alone after the baby was born. Once the baby was born, we would want our chance to grieve, and we wanted that grief to be private.

On the morning of the interviews my already fragile state of mind was further shaken by the news of the article quoting the Diocese about our situation. I was feeling disappointed and angry about the Church's statement as I rushed around my bedroom trying to ready myself for the events of the day. Before I ran out the door I took a blood pressure reading, and as the cuff released its grip on my arm, I glanced at the reading and did a double-take. It was significantly high. I knew I couldn't call the doctor because the office wasn't open yet. *This could be the day*, I thought. Dr. Read had indicated that all she needed was to hear of fluctuating pressures, and she'd deliver. I knew this was her surgery day, so she'd be in the hospital and could easily slip me into her schedule.

I took a few deep breaths and took my pressure again. The next reading was better. I got my bag for the hospital and checked to see if everything was inside. We'd been going to the hospital so many times in the previous few weeks that I wasn't sure if all the items were still in place. As I checked the bag, I looked up and out the window of our bedroom—this same bedroom where I'd first heard the news seven months earlier and run from one side of it to the other trying to escape the reality of what was about to happen to us. Here we were at the other side of a painful journey, but we'd made it. The baby was healthy, our marriage was strong, and we had our own baby on the way. I thought back to the morning of February 16, when I lay in my bed content that I was pregnant. I was thrilled that a new baby would be joining our family. I never could have imagined what that day and these past seven months had in store for us. Now I stood and stared out the same window. It was a beautiful crisp fall day, with clear skies. The leaves on the trees had just started to turn. This would be a perfect day for Little Man to enter our world.

I picked up my hospital bag when my mom came in.

"What's going on?"

"We're going to the hospital right after the press thing," I said.

"What? Are you sure that makes sense, Carolyn? I mean, if you need to go to the hospital, you should probably go right away," she said, a worried frown on her face.

"Mom, I'm okay," I said. "I just had a blood pressure spike. I'm not in any danger. But I am preparing to be admitted. That does not necessarily mean delivery."

"I'll call your father," she said. "If he leaves from Michigan now, he'll get here before the baby is born."

"Don't do that yet. Wait until I call you after I speak to Dr. Read," I said and headed out the door.

At the PR firm, the television crews from the various local stations were in each of the four conference rooms. Every fifteen minutes, we moved to meet with a different crew. We finished our interviews right on schedule. I called Dr. Read's nurse, who, as expected, sent us straight to labor and delivery.

"Does that mean we are doing the C-section today?" Sean asked.

"No. We have to get to the hospital and wait to see what Dr. Read says. I assume she'll want to run some tests."

"Should we call Shannon and Paul?" Sean asked.

"Not yet. Let's wait until we know what's going to happen."

Sean dropped me off at the visitors' entrance, and I walked right past admitting and straight up to the maternity floor. I checked in at the nurses' station and found a friendly and familiar face waiting for me.

"We heard you were coming in, so I called dibs!" It was Colleen, my nurse from MK's delivery, who had since become a friend.

"Great. Have you heard from Dr. Read?"

"Yup. We are doing it today. Three P.M."

I stopped dead in my tracks.

"Really?"

"Really. Are you ready?"

Was I ready to say hello and good-bye to my baby? How could I be ready for that? But I would honor this child. I would demonstrate our love for him today. We had done everything we could to prepare for this moment. I nodded to Colleen, picked up my phone, and started to inform everyone else who needed to prepare.

My first call had to be Shannon. I'd felt so dumb for calling her the other night with a false alarm and getting her all excited. She'd arranged for the care of her girls, only to get a call from Sean less than an hour later to report that I'd been discharged. I swore I'd never alarm her again unless I was certain, and now the certainty had arrived.

"Shannon, we're having the baby today," I said.

"Really? When?"

"Dr. Read is going to do the C-section at three o'clock. Can you get here by then?" It was 11:30 A.M., so I thought they could make it.

"Don't wait for us. If they have to do it now, don't wait for us."

"We will wait for you. That's not a problem."

"Okay. Well, I was supposed to get my hair done and then give an interview to Fox National at 1:00 P.M. I guess I could cancel the hair appointment, pull my hair back in a ponytail, and do the interview and just leave straight from there?"

"Okay."

"Well, I don't want to cancel because I don't want them to know the baby is coming today."

"I get it. Do what you need to do. We'll wait."

"Okay. I think we'll be there in time. This is so exciting!"

I could hear the joy in her voice. I hung up the phone chuckling to myself about Shannon frantically running around trying to figure out how to wear her hair. She was clearly excited!

I made the rest of my calls. My neighbor would care for the kids, my mom and dad were en route, JoAnn was also coming to pray and boss people around (which I asked her to do), and my friend

Kathleen was coming with her camera to document the delivery. That was it. No one else was to be told where we were. We didn't want a soul to learn that Little Man was here until we knew he was healthy and safely at home with Paul and Shannon. We'd even made arrangements for the Morells to get their own room in the NICU because it is a very secure place. Only people who were buzzed in by the staff could enter.

I had an alias, Diane Strick, which was also on my hospital wristband. The hospital provided us with security guards who only allowed those who knew my alias to come in contact with me. We were also concerned that the Morells might be mobbed by the press if they set up outside the hospital. The hospital arranged for them to park their car away from the normal hospital parking lot in a place where they would be greeted by the head of the hospital team.

By 2:00 P.M., my family and friends had arrived. They all sat around my bed, and we laughed and talked together. It was a new experience for me. I had never entered into a delivery feeling so healthy. As the Morells arrived, Shannon called me.

"Carolyn?" Shannon was crying.

"Are you okay? Are you crying?"

"I want you there when we meet the baby. I think you should be there."

I was touched by her offer.

"That's very sweet of you, Shannon. But I can't be there. I have to stay in the OR and get sewn up. Sean will come. Is that okay?"

"I really think you should both be there. But yes, that will do."

I hung up and appreciated the gesture.

Once we knew the Morells had arrived at the hospital, Dr. Read said it was time.

"Do you want a wheelchair?" Colleen asked.

"I don't really need one," I said. "I'm not sick."

"If you want to, you can walk," Colleen offered.

"I can?" I asked, delighted. My previous births were such madness. I'd had to be wheeled in on a gurney in an atmosphere of disaster.

"That's what most women do when they are having a scheduled C-section," Colleen said.

As I stood up, a big grin spread over my face. I would walk into the delivery room with my head held high. This was going to be a beautiful birth to honor my precious Little Man.

I turned to say good-bye to my family. We all hugged, and the last in line was my dad. He held me tight in a great big bear hug and whispered in my ear.

"I love you, sugar. We are so proud of you," my dad said.

I knew he was. I knew they all were. I winked back at him and smiled. I had made my daddy proud, and there's only goodness in that.

As I walked down the hallway it was like a parade. I was with Dr. Read and the security guard, plus Kathleen, Colleen, and some of the other people who would be assisting in the C-section.

As we walked past the nurses' station, they all stood up, as if in respect.

The operating room was very cold, and I shivered as I lay down. Sean came in all suited up in hospital scrubs and took my hand as they raised the drape between my chest and lower body so that I couldn't see the C-section. The room was crowded. There was a team from the NICU to evaluate the baby, including a nurse-practitioner I remembered from Mary Kate's birth. Dr. Read had asked another surgeon to attend the delivery because she wanted to be careful about any problems with the placenta, which was still sitting very low in my uterus. Plus there was the anesthesiologist and his nurse. Quite a party.

I was concerned about the spinal because the one I'd had when Mary Kate was born wasn't very good. I felt a lot more of that procedure than I thought I should. As the anesthesiologist tapped into the base of my spine and I felt the drug spreading through my nervous system, I didn't think he'd given me enough.

"I can still move my toes," I advised him.

"We're not operating on your toes," the anesthesiologist said.

"Well, I'm glad we cleared that up," I joked.

I looked at Sean, so funny in his puffy surgical hat. He held my hand just like he had that night we met, when we walked through campus. Here we were, twenty years later, in this unbelievable situation. How could we have known when we were that young how severely life would test us? Sean had protected us so well. We could focus completely on this moment. Maybe there would be horrible emotions on the other side of this delivery, but for this instant we could appreciate all that we'd been through to bring this life into the world.

As soon as they started to cut me open, I felt nauseous. The anesthesiologist was quick to give me something for that so I wouldn't miss anything. I felt the tugging and pulling that I remembered from MK's delivery. The rearranging of my insides and the feeling of all those hands inside of me was awful, but it was mercifully quick.

"We are taking the baby out now!"

I shut my eyes and felt the pressure that I had carried for the past eight months lift off of my chest as my lungs reinflated. In a matter of moments, I heard Little Man take his first breath in our world and let out a huge yell. He was the feisty little guy who had been doing back flips in my womb.

"Do you want to see him?" one of the nurses asked.

Of course, I thought. I later thought they were probably trying to be sensitive to me by asking. Perhaps, like a woman who is going to have her baby adopted by another couple, I might not want to see him.

"Yes, yes," I said. "Of course I do."

One of the NICU nurses brought him around the drape, and I

saw him all pink and covered in goop. He looked huge! So much bigger than Mary Kate and Ryan had been. They rushed him into a room to my right to evaluate him as Kathleen snapped dozens of pictures. After a few minutes, they brought him back to me swaddled in a blanket and wearing a little newborn cap.

"His APGAR score is a nine on a scale of ten," the nurse reported. "And his lungs are working beautifully."

Yes!

Exactly what we'd hoped, planned, and prayed for.

A few minutes passed before a nurse came over and placed our tightly swaddled infant in Sean's arms. I looked up at Sean's face and saw that he was crying as he studied Little Man. I think his tears were tears of joy, but for me, my joy resulted in a smile. I was thrilled.

Sean held him as close to me as he could, since the continued surgery was keeping me restricted. I kissed Little Man on the top of his head and laughed with elation as he opened his eyes and looked right into my face.

"Hi, Little Man. Hi, sweetie."

I said this again as I took off his cap to get a good look at that magnificent head of hair that we'd seen so many times in the ultrasounds. He looked perfect. I put my face up against his and kissed him over and over. He was born at 3:18 P.M., and we had only a few minutes with him before Sean had to take him down to the Morells. I was nauseous again, and they gave me another shot of something to help me as Sean walked the baby over to the nurses, who placed him in an isolette for his journey to meet his parents.

The idea that the baby I had just delivered had to go meet his parents was still such a confusing thought for me. I knew that until that moment when they cut the umbilical cord, he was my baby. In those moments in the delivery room, he still felt like he was ours. I had the pride of a mother at childbirth, and I had all the love. No matter how we'd prepared, in the moment it was incredible to me that I couldn't keep this baby. There were many who believd he'd never really been mine, but I knew that, until the moment when they took him out of that room and down the hall, he still was.

"How much does he weigh?" I asked.

The NICU staff was so caught up in the moment that they hadn't weighed him. They had to take all his blankets off and place him on the scale.

"Five pounds, three ounces!"

Wow. He was a whopper at four weeks early. They wrapped him up again. I looked at him as completely as I could, my heart open to our little miracle, our lucky little boy.

"Shall we take him now?" one of the nurses asked.

No, don't take him. Let me keep him. He belongs with our family. His rightful place is in my arms. He is a part of me.

"Yes. Take him. Go, go, go," I said. "Take him."

CHAPTER 19

A Broken Hallelujah

SEAN

I HELD CAROLYN'S HAND with my left hand while wiping away a tear of joy with my right hand. I leaned down really close to her ear and whispered, "I love you." I kissed her cheek. What Carolyn had done was beautiful, and the baby that the nurses wrapped snugly in receiving blankets seemed like a gift to the world from God. To see him with Carolyn, to hold him for just a moment, was an honor. I was living literally second by second, holding on to every detail. I knew that for that brief time, and for that time only, he was ours. We might see him again. We might even be allowed to kiss him and hug him, but after this moment we would need permission to do so.

Carolyn was pale and shaky. So much of me wanted to stay by her side and hold her hand through the next difficult part of the surgery, but I felt what can only be described as a deep calling to deliver this beautiful child to his genetic parents.

Ever since we entered the second trimester I'd feared this moment. I felt fear now, and pain and anger were nearby. But those feelings were balanced by a powerful feeling of love, the same love we'd felt as the baby grew inside Carolyn, but now it seemed to touch every molecule of the air around us. And it was so clear that Carolyn's incredible act of sacrifice throughout the long eight months needed to be honored. The dignified way to transition this baby from the Savage family to the Morell family was in person. I could feel the love softening into surrender and a willingness to let him go. I hadn't expected this, but I welcomed it.

Carolyn has always said that the greatest joy of giving a gift is watching the recipient unwrap it. I would be her eyes and ears as the Morells received this ultimate gift. I also wanted Paul and Shannon to see with their own eyes that other human beings were delivering their child: he didn't just miraculously fall from the sky. This wasn't an abstraction. By seeing the pain in my eyes, I hoped they'd have a window into the loss that Carolyn and I were experiencing and accept the child in the spirit in which we were giving him.

"Sean, are you ready?" a nurse asked.

I nodded yes. I took one more glance at my beautiful wife and watched as they placed the baby in the isolette. A nurse pushed him toward the exit doors, and I fell in line behind.

In the hallway, a security guard led the procession. I stood directly behind the isolette, with a nurse on the left guiding it and another nurse on the right. Our friend Kathleen trailed behind with her camera. The hospital had planned a route that took us down cold and dimly lit corridors with concrete floors and stark white walls. The public didn't have access to these hallways, and we saw no one else on our walk down to the elevators. We walked slowly, silently, and in a mood of perfect reverence.

As I looked inside the isolette, I saw the baby's arms moving and his eyes opening and closing, the signs of a soul awakening to the world, trying to take it all in. A powerful mix of emotions penetrated me: deep sorrow and mourning, but at the same time great satisfaction that we'd gotten to this point and given this child life. I thought of songwriter Leonard Cohen's words "a broken hallelujah." Each step of our walk contained a hallelujah of praise and thanksgiving for this child wrapped in the broken feeling of the impending loss. As we approached the elevator, suddenly I felt a penetrating pain throughout my body, and I began to shake. The security guard punched the button, and the elevator seemed to take forever to come to our floor. I would have been happy to wait forever to extend my time with the baby.

We exited on the NICU floor, the same floor where the Morells waited, and took a circuitous route through the lonely corridors. My tears flowed as they had since we exited the labor and delivery room. I didn't care that I was crying. It helped that I could feel the profound respect of everyone I was with. It genuinely felt like they were suffering for and with me.

As we approached the NICU, I felt a rush of adrenaline pumping into my bloodstream. I knew that I needed to muster the spirit to celebrate with Paul and Shannon. I knew they would be thrilled, thankful beyond description, and I wanted to be with them in their happiness.

We entered the double doors to the NICU, doors I'd been through a hundred times in the month after Mary Kate's birth. I recognized many of the staff, who stood in silence. They all knew what I was about to do.

We stood for just a moment outside the room where Paul and Shannon waited for this "second delivery" of their son.

Please, God, let me get through this, I prayed.

One of the nurses opened the door as we moved into the room.

I saw Shannon first, standing at the back of the room, with Paul behind her. I don't think the staff had given the Morells any warning that we were coming.

Shannon shrieked with joy and clapped her hands together as I pushed the baby into the room. She pointed at the baby in disbelief, exclaiming, "Oh, my God! Oh, my God! Oh, my God!" as she jumped up and down, clenching her hands to her chest.

"Congratulations, you have a healthy baby boy. Five pounds, three ounces," I announced.

"I can't believe it! I can't believe it! He is really here!" she cried out. She had her hands on her cheeks. I had expected that they would be joyful, yet thankful and respectful. Her response took me off-guard.

Paul came to the isolette smiling, and Shannon followed. They stood beside it looking down at their baby boy. I smiled for them. At that moment, the nurse behind me placed a soft hand on my shoulder. It was like the touch of an angel, a kind spirit who had just made the walk with me, acknowledging my suffering. She whispered in my ear, "This must be so hard for you." Another big tear rolled down my cheek as I shook my head yes.

"Shannon, do you want to hold the baby?" another nurse asked.

"Can I? Can I!!?"

"Yes," the nurse said as she gingerly took the baby out of the isolette and handed him to Shannon.

I put aside my sorrow and felt the happiness of seeing a baby held by his mom and then his dad for the first time. Shannon spoke to the baby softly, but I couldn't hear her words.

Shannon and Paul wanted to get a few photographs, but they said that their camera wasn't working. I asked Kathleen to take some pictures. The Morells invited me to be in a few. I was pleased to participate. My swollen eyes would just have to be part of the picture, as it would take hours for them to look normal again.

I didn't want to stay too long.

"I should get going and give you time alone," I said.

"Sean, one minute," Shannon said. She motioned me over. "We want to tell you his name, but please don't tell anyone but Carolyn."

"No problem."

"His name is Logan Savage Morell. Logan for 'lucky,' because when we first met you, you said we were lucky. Savage because Savage is my maiden name and your last names."

I didn't remember telling them they were lucky, but I appreciated the sentiment.

"I think that's neat, Shannon, and I'm sure Carolyn will be

pleased. Congratulations again," I said. "I'm going to leave now. I need to see how Carolyn is doing."

When I walked out of the room, I felt the wind sucked out of me. I stood in the silent hallway for a moment. Everything that had just happened seemed like a blur. Everyone who'd accompanied me appeared frozen. I walked out of the NICU and into the hallway, heading toward the elevator alone. This was the moment I had previously envisioned when I would punch a hole through the wall. That feeling never came. Instead, I felt despair. My hands were empty. The broken hallelujah was all I had.

I went back to the elevator to return to the maternity floor, but I was in no-man's-land. I didn't know where to go or what to do. I was surprised that Carolyn wasn't yet in the recovery room. One of the nurses said that she was still in the delivery room. I wanted to be with Carolyn so much. Instead, I walked into the room where JoAnn was waiting with Carolyn's parents and updated them.

"The baby was five pounds, three ounces. He is doing really well. Carolyn did well," I announced.

"Are you doing okay?" Carolyn's father asked.

"No, not at all," I struggled to get out. Probably for the first time in my life I wanted out of my own skin.

I needed to get out of there and find Carolyn. I wondered how she could still be in surgery. Why was it taking so long for them to let me see her? I walked the hall to try to find a place to myself. What the hell was I supposed to do? In our normal birth situation, I would be with Carolyn, rifling off celebratory calls and text messages to my family and friends, announcing the birth. Instead, I was in the corner of a hallway with my back against the wall. I slid down the wall until I was sitting on the floor and buried my face in my hands. What was going on? I looked up to see a security guard watching over me. What must be going through his head right now?

More time passed. I realized that I didn't know how to handle my grief without Carolyn. I didn't have anyone to talk to about my worries about her health or my feelings about the scene with the Morells and the baby.

Then I really started to worry. What if something had gone terribly wrong with the delivery after I left? That seemed so impossible because she was conscious and talking when I last saw her.

Finally, Dr. Read appeared.

"Sean, Carolyn is going to be up shortly. After you left, she started bleeding, and we couldn't stop it," Dr. Read said. "We lost track of how much blood she lost. I am very thankful that the other surgeon was there because we both had to work independently to help Carolyn. It was one of the most difficult deliveries I've ever done."

My throat went dry, and I could not speak for a moment. All that time I was walking the halls desperate to see Carolyn, she was in terrible danger. On the one hand, I wish I had been with her. On the other hand, it all seemed too much to bear to think that Carolyn's health had been compromised. I felt so thankful to the medical team.

"Dr. Read, thank you so much for getting her through," I said. "We cannot thank you enough."

"We will monitor her closely in the event that she needs a transfusion," Dr. Read said. "She is going to be very weak. I am going home this evening, but they can call me at a moment's notice."

After she left, those words "one of the most difficult deliveries" stayed in my mind. Suddenly my memory was thrown back to Ryan's delivery twelve years earlier, which had also been frightening. Then the enormity of the fact that Carolyn nearly lost everything for this baby boy really hit me. I was sick to my stomach. I prayed with all I had for Carolyn to be all right. I needed to be able to call the boys and tell them their mom was okay. *I* needed her to be okay. Was this too much to ask?

Within minutes, thank God, Carolyn arrived in recovery, pale, weak, and just strong enough to say a few words.

"Carolyn, you're so strong," I said as I leaned down to kiss her. "Everything is going to be all right. It's all going to be fine."

I didn't believe my own words, but I had to reassure her. Carolyn, heavily medicated, drifted off to sleep, but I couldn't. I sat by her bed and watched her.

Later that evening, as Carolyn slept, I called my mom to update her and then Marty, who knew we were in the hospital. I decided to call our publicist in New York, who also knew we were in the hospital. I wanted to make sure he did not worry about us overnight. In confidence, I let him know of the delivery and medical status. I instructed him not to release this information to anyone in the media. As I hung up, just to be crystal clear, I sent him an e-mail from my BlackBerry, restating my instruction that he was not to release the birth information to anyone in the media. He responded right away with "I understand."

I finally drifted off to sleep, but slept only fitfully. I kept waking up to make sure that Carolyn was all right. At one point I jolted awake with repeated visions of walking through the doorway to hand Logan to Paul and Shannon. Then I realized, with a combination of some relief and great pain, that that moment had passed.

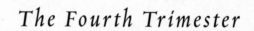

The Fourth Trimester

CHAPTER 20

Wrapped in Love

CAROLYN

I WOKE UP the next day feeling weak and thickheaded from the painkillers. Despite the morphine, I could feel the ache in the place where Logan used to be. Logan. Little Man's name was Logan. I remembered seeing him as he kicked and screamed moments after he was born. Logan was a great name for my feisty Little Man. It had an old-fashioned, romantic sound to it. Would all the girls swoon for Logan? I hoped I'd be around to find out.

In the hours after each of my children were born, my mind was full of fantasies of the great lives they would live, and the morning after Logan's birth was no different. I hoped he'd be a boy with many friends. I pictured him shooting hoops with Drew and Ryan. *Stop that, Carolyn. You don't know that he'll take up that sport or any sport at all.* Another image quickly replaced that one: of Logan on his hands and knees crawling rapid-fire into the family room and pulling himself up, hand over hand, on the big leather chair. *Oh, Carolyn, you're just torturing yourself.* Yet it was so easy for me to picture him in our home. I honestly couldn't picture him anywhere else. When they placed Logan on my chest in the delivery room, I had stared at his face and thought how much he looked like Drew.

If we hadn't known about the mistake, we would never have figured it out on our own.

The door swung open, and Sue, one my favorite nurses, entered. She didn't look happy.

"Mrs. Savage, I came to tell you that the baby is being released today," she said. "He's well enough, and they want to go home," she said.

"What?" I tried to sit up, but my stitches wouldn't let me. I had bled so much that a drain had to be placed in my wound, and that was causing me even more pain than my previous C-sections. I was panicking.

"They're going to let me see him, right?" I asked. "They're not leaving right now? I so want the kids to meet him."

"No. They said you could have some time with him this afternoon," she said.

I knew he'd be leaving more quickly than Ryan and MK had, but in less than twenty-four hours?

"Are you sure? I mean, I'm so out of it," I said. "I want to be able to spend time with him. I want to memorize his face. I can hardly focus my eyes!"

"If you want to be lucid, you need to turn off your morphine pump," Sue advised. "Then we can get you into the shower and pretty you up for some pictures. We'll move you to a larger room where you can get some photographs of your time with him and all your family."

I knew she was right about what I should do to prepare, but I was only sixteen hours postsurgery. Still, I couldn't miss this.

"Turn off the morphine pump and I'll deal."

About thirty minutes later, JoAnn arrived. She and Sue hoisted me out of my bed, and I tottered to the shower. I was extremely light-headed, and I could feel that I was still bleeding. As I stood in the shower, JoAnn held my clothes and a towel, while Sue hosed me off like an elephant at the circus. To think I used to be such a modest and private person before this pregnancy.

After the shower, I began to feel a little more human. Sue moved me down the hallway to a room big enough to have two entrances. One wall had windows overlooking the trees of west Toledo, brilliant in their fall colors. I'd just settled in when Sean's mom Kate arrived. I think of Kate as my second mother, and as a great friend. Seeing her got my mind off what was about to happen.

A few minutes later, Sean arrived, along with my mom, Drew, Ryan, and Mary Kate. As soon as Mary Kate saw me, her smile spread from ear to ear. She practically dove into my bed. I wrapped my arms around her and snuggled her close, feeling maternal hunger throughout my body. I needed a baby to snuggle, and my eighteen-month-old daughter would have to be the one.

Sean snapped a few pictures of MK and me, and Kate started to gather her things.

"Are you leaving, Kate?" I asked.

"Oh, yes," Kate said. "I know they are bringing the baby up, and I want to give you all your private time."

"But, Kate, you don't have to leave."

"You know, I appreciate that. I really do. The truth is, I don't think I can watch this." She was tearing up. "I'm afraid it is just too hard for me. I don't want to see the baby."

I understood. Kate had borne nine children. She had prayed relentlessly for Sean and me during our years of infertility. This was a good-bye too difficult for her to witness.

"Please come back later," I said. "I'd like to have you here."

Before she could answer, the security guard opened the main door.

"They're bringing the baby down the hall," she said.

Kate looked horrified, and I held up my hand.

"Hold on. Kate would like to leave before you bring the baby in. Just one minute," I said.

As they pushed Logan's isolette in, Kate slid out the second door, timing her movements carefully to avoid seeing him in the hallway.

Sue rolled the isolette to me, and the six of us crowded around to marvel at Logan.

"Everyone, I want you to meet Logan Savage Morell," Sue said as she lifted him up and placed him in my arms. I caught the faces of the boys and my mom. I would have never known, in that moment, that they weren't looking at their new baby brother and grandson.

"Hrmph."

"What, Mary Kate?"

She had clearly said something, but I had no idea what. When I twisted around to look at her, I noticed that her sweet little face was all pinched up as if she had tasted something sour.

"Do you see the baby? Isn't he cute, Mary Kate?"

She looked away.

"I don't think she likes him, Mom," Ryan said.

My baby girl was horrified that her mommy had another baby in her arms. She wanted nothing to do with a new infant. I handed Logan to Ryan, who is a natural with babies. He peered at Logan and ever so gently rocked him. By this time, Mary Kate had thrown herself on the ground in a tantrum. Ryan handed Logan to Drew, who was less comfortable holding babies. When Ryan placed Logan in Drew's arms, Drew's whole body tightened, but he smiled. My mom held him next. Sean was snapping pictures fast, trying to get every angle.

The whole visit was only thirty minutes so that Sean and I could have some time alone with Logan before we returned him to the Morells. But first, we wanted a family picture with Logan. Sean stood next to me holding Mary Kate. Drew and Ryan stood behind us on either side. My mom snapped a few quick photos in the moments when Mary Kate wasn't squirming and complaining. By the end of the session, she'd calmed down and could even muster a wisp of a smile. Then it was time for the boys and Mary Kate to say good-bye to Logan. Drew and Ryan took one last look and walked out of the room with Grandma Linda and Mary Kate.

"I am so glad we had them come," Sean said.

"I loved seeing the boys hold Logan," I said.

I laid Logan on my lap and carefully unwrapped his blanket so that I could slide him out of his T-shirt to look at his little body.

"We did that! He is perfect," I said, joyfully.

"No, Carolyn. You did that. And he is perfect," Sean said.

I held him up and turned him around, inspecting his little arms, fingers, chest, and toes. We had seen his tiny body so many times in the black-and-white images of the ultrasounds, but it was nice to get a good look at him.

He was getting a bit upset at being exposed, so I quickly laid him on his belly on top of my chest. Instinctively, he snuggled his head under my chin and immediately quieted himself. Within a few seconds, he closed his eyes and slept in the crook of my neck.

"He can probably hear your heartbeat," Sean said. "He's listened to it all these months. It stopped him from crying, you know?"

The second I laid him down and his face rested against my skin, I knew. He knew. I had felt this feeling before, with my other three, but this time. . . . How could that feeling be there? How could this feel so right? How could he be theirs? He felt like mine.

He is yours. He is theirs. He is God's gift to all of us.

As I held Logan on my chest, I heard the familiar ping of a text message arriving on my BlackBerry. I picked it up, flung it open, and stared at its contents. Jennifer had been to an appointment and sent me an ultrasound picture. I stared at my baby and rubbed the back of Logan. Two precious lives that I loved more than I could express. I felt lucky in that moment.

After a few minutes of cuddling, I turned him on his back and swaddled him tightly. I stared at his tiny face as he slept peacefully in my arms.

"Look here, Little Man. You can't just leave us. You have to pull some strings for us with your mommy and daddy. We want to see you. We want to watch you grow. So, if you use your pull right, we'll see you so often you'll think we are related."

Logan opened his eyes and looked right at me. I couldn't believe what I was seeing. I think he understood, and as our eyes locked I could feel his soul. I knew then that we'd always be connected.

SEAN

As CAROLYN HELD LOGAN to her chest, I could barely contain my emotion. Fifteen hours before, she had held him inside her, now she was holding him on her chest, and a few hours from now he would be gone with the Morells in Michigan. How could we pack a lifetime of love for this child into a few minutes?

Carolyn handed Logan to me. I cuddled him in my arms and sat in the rocking chair. I had a bottle for him, and I gently rocked him while he ate. As I was holding Logan, he was in and out of sleep. I was so relaxed and one with him, just as I had been with Drew, Ryan, and Mary Kate. Carolyn could barely move, because of the pain, but she pulled herself out of bed, and the nurse took dozens of pictures of Carolyn, Logan, and me. As I held him I watched the clock, knowing that our time with him was quickly coming to an end.

Just then, Sue came in to ask us something she and the other nurses wanted to know.

"Would you want me to do a bereavement box?" she said. "We do these for families who lose a child at or after birth."

Carolyn and I looked at each other, pained that this was the appropriate gesture to make for a baby who at that moment was resting so sweetly in my arms.

"Yes," I said softly.

Moments later she came in with the box. She held one of Logan's feet to make an imprint of it in clay. Next, she took our picture, hustled down the hall to get it printed, and then placed it in the box along with other personal items. When she brought the box back, she placed it on a shelf. As she shut the door she said, "I will leave you two alone with the baby for your remaining time."

I stared at the box, and then back at Logan, and then again at the box. I didn't know what we would do with it, but I was thankful to Sue and her team for recognizing our loss.

I wanted Carolyn to be the last to hold him. I helped her move the four feet from her bed to the rocker. She grimaced as she sat in the chair, but she wanted to rock Logan so badly. I handed Logan to her.

"He is so beautiful and so alert," I said.

"It feels so good to have some time to simply focus on him and put everything else aside."

I took pictures from every angle. Next, I grabbed the video camera and recorded a brief moment. Carolyn smiled in a way that I had not seen her smile this year. She was captured by Logan.

Sue rolled the isolette back in, and we knew what that meant: Paul and Shannon were coming to get Logan. It was time to say good-bye. We had done everything we could in forty-five minutes. As Carolyn placed him in the isolette, we held his hand and leaned in to kiss him on the forehead, saying, "I love you."

After Logan had left, I helped Carolyn back into bed, and Mary Smith arrived. She carried with her a thick stack of documents and her notary seal, the paperwork to officially turn custody of Logan over to the Morells.

Mary had a pen for each of us. One by one, she handed us the documents, explaining the reason for each one. I heard her, but I did not listen. For the only time in my life, I signed legal documents that I didn't read. I knew that the cold, dry wording on these papers could not reflect the love we were feeling for Logan. The papers had to say that we didn't want to be his parents, and I just could not read such wording. Carolyn and I signed our names again and again and again. The few pictures we took of that moment when we signed away our formal connection to Logan reflect our reluctant surrender. We were fulfilling our commitment, and it felt like hell.

Mary brought all of the signed documents to Shannon and Paul. After they signed off, she drove to the Lucas County courthouse, where a judge made the change of custody final. We officially lost Logan with the drop of a gavel at a courthouse just one mile from the hospital at 4:00 P.M. on September 25, 2009. From that moment, we knew we could never go back.

The New York public relations person proved to be untrustworthy. I had been clear in my messages to him that we did not want news of the birth to be released. He released the news anyway, and word spread quickly. Calls were coming in nonstop to me and family members as well as to our attorneys and the local PR firm. Carolyn and I terminated our relationship with the New York PR firm that day, deciding that we could get all the expertise we needed from our local firm. The media pressure grew to a frenzy as the day went on. We decided to put together a joint statement with the Morells, hoping that that would satisfy the media.

As the day progressed I jotted down some thoughts, and the Morells had ideas about their statement. In the afternoon, we realized that it would be difficult for the two families to speak as one. Their experience was vastly different from ours. It was impossible to issue a joint statement that captured their celebration and our loss. We agreed to release separate statements once the Morells had left the hospital with Logan.

The last step we would take before saying a final good-bye was to write notes for Logan. As I put pen to paper I chose my words carefully, knowing that Logan might not read this letter for many years.

Carolyn and I wanted Logan to know that our choice to let him go was the highest form of love we could give. As a caterpillar comes out of his cocoon and becomes the butterfly, Logan was flying away from us, but our love, hopes, and dreams for him would remain within us forever. I prayed that someday he would read these letters that said, even though we were far away, we would always think of him and always love him.

The nurse opened our door to say, "I understand the Morells are getting ready to leave. If you want to see them, I suggest that you head down to their room."

She must have received a call from a nurse in the NICU. It was about 6:45, just twenty-seven hours after delivery.

"Sean, we need to say good-bye and give him the chest of gifts we bought," Carolyn said.

"Okay, let's go!"

I pushed Carolyn to the elevator in a wheelchair and then down the hall to the NICU into Paul and Shannon's room. Paul held Logan as Shannon gathered up their things. They knew we were coming, but were understandably eager to leave.

"Please sit down," Shannon said.

"We have some gifts for Logan and for you," Carolyn said.

"Oh, you shouldn't have. You don't need to give us anything," Shannon said.

"We wanted him to have certain things," I commented.

Carolyn handed Shannon the treasure chest that we had filled with some gifts. We hoped Logan would someday cherish and understand the meaning behind each item we chose.

Shannon sat in a chair across from Carolyn talking about the media inquiries that were pouring into her cell phone. Carolyn nodded as if she was listening, but I don't think either of us was paying any attention. I could see Carolyn's eyes drifting over to the corner of the room, where Paul stood with his back to us, holding Logan. We were both trying to steal our last glimpses of the baby.

As the moments passed, things became awkward. Our presence in the room started to feel like an intrusion. Carolyn and I wished them well. I patted Logan on his head as we turned to exit. They would be on the road within minutes.

We stepped out into the hallway. As the door to their room slammed behind us, we froze for a few seconds in silence. I pushed the wheelchair closer to Carolyn, and she sat. We made our way into our room at about 7:15. I had a cold feeling. What should we do now? Carolyn sat in her bed, and I sat next to her and put my arm around her, and we wept. As Paul and Shannon drove away with Logan in a car seat, we wept. As the world moved on, we wept.

CHAPTER 21

Good-byes and Grief

CAROLYN

THREE DAYS POSTDELIVERY, I was thrilled to be going home, but dreading how I would feel leaving the hospital with empty arms. During the pregnancy, our days had been so full. I had included the baby growing inside me in every thought. He helped me decide if I should lift something and when I needed to let the housework go. I'd always decided my social calendar with him in mind. He even showed me what to eat. Besides the ache in my heart and the scar across my belly, would his departure leave a lot of free space in my mind? I wouldn't be dreaming about or fearing what it would be like at the birth or when we left him with his parents. That was all done now, and my images of it were strong. Only time would show me what those memories meant to me. Would they be good ones of a time when Sean and I rose to do the right thing on a unique occasion? Or would I always think of this experience only as a loss?

I knew that the gap would have more dimensions than just the absence of Logan. Sean and I had become so close in this crisis. I would always be grateful to him for the way he sheltered me and left nothing to chance. He's not a man who is comfortable with emotion, but he walked right into the fire holding my hand. Yes, we fought, but it was always as two people who were completely committed, both to each other and to making the best of whatever life brought our way. During this crisis, we were on the phone to each other multiple times a day. As things settled, would I miss Sean too? There was no way of knowing what faced me at my house, which now somehow seemed filled with empty rooms.

Dr. Read came to see me shortly before I left. She sat on my bed. I'd never seen that look on her face before. She had been my savior throughout this pregnancy, and she never lost her professional demeanor. As she looked into my eyes, her expression was gentle. I felt the compassion that came from her very core, the kindness in her heart that made her a healer.

"I'm worried, Carolyn," she said. "I've sent patients home from the hospital after tragedies before. But this is different. What can I do to help you?"

"Remember in July when I told you I was afraid of postpartum depression? Well, I think it's here. I didn't sleep last night. I doubt I'll sleep soundly for a very long time. I'm afraid of what the darkness and quiet of night will bring me."

Dr. Read took a pen and paper from the pocket of her doctor's coat and wrote down the number of Linda Vanderpol, a therapist.

"Call her. I'll call her too. Bereavement after the loss of a newborn is her specialty. I'll let her know that you need to be seen immediately," she said. "If she thinks you need something to help you, then I'll prescribe it."

She handed me the paper and grabbed my hands. "You did a wonderful thing. You know that, right? I've seen a lot of things in my career, but nothing as special as this. It was a privilege to be a part of this journey."

She was crying. I was crying and couldn't find any words. I shook my head yes and looked back at the floor. I was so lucky she was my doctor.

"Dr. Read, there is one thing you can do. Could you please do something about these?"

I pointed at my swollen chest, and she laughed out of sympathy.

"No. Not a thing I can do about that. When the milk comes in, do not express any, and you'll dry out in a few days. In the meantime, wear two bras and take some ibuprofen."

After she left, I quickly packed my bags, and one of the nuns, who was also a nurse, helped me pile the dozens of gifts that had arrived at the hospital during my stay on a cart so that we could bring them down to the car. I asked her if she could distribute some of the flower arrangements I had received from the media and well-wishers I had never met to other patients. I couldn't imagine taking them all home.

The nun placed them on another cart and walked out of the room to start delivering them. A few seconds after she left, I realized that I had accidentally left a gift bag from the Reliable Girls on the cart. I bolted out of my room and sprinted down the hall. I saw her waiting at the elevator.

"Wow, I didn't know you could move that fast," the nun said.

"There it is," I said, pointing to a bag on one of the lower shelves. I didn't want to stretch my stitches by reaching down to pick it up.

The nun grabbed the gift bag to hand it to me, and as she lifted it, out slid a super-size bottle of Ketel One.

"Is this what you wanted?"

I wrapped my hand around the neck of the bottle and said, "Yup. That's what I want."

She looked me directly in the eye.

"Oh, don't worry. I won't open it until I'm at home."

She giggled like a schoolgirl, and I turned on my heels and marched back to my room with a bottle of vodka in one hand and a bottle of Apple Pucker in the other. I doubted I'd be mixing an appletini that night, but I had been on the wagon for nine long months, and if any event warranted a cocktail, this was it.

Soon after that, Sean and the kids arrived to take me home. My nurse brought me a wheelchair, and I gingerly put my feet on the footrests.

Shouldn't I be holding a baby? I thought to myself.

It was the third time in my life I had left the hospital after delivery without an infant in my arms, and I was sad.

If you want to hold a baby, then hold a baby!

I turned around and motioned to Sean to give me Mary Kate. He handed her over, and she snuggled in my arms. Drew and Ryan walked beside me while Sean went ahead to bring the car around. As we walked out of my hospital room, I felt strong and courageous. I was lifted by the presence of my three children.

As we rolled by the nurses' station, I was surprised to find a crowd of a dozen nurses, Dr. Read, and a few other hospital employees. They handed me a card they had all signed that said how privileged they felt to have been part of this event. I thanked them. I couldn't have chosen a better group of professionals to be involved in our care.

That night, before I went to bed, I checked my e-mail, hoping for a message about Logan. I hadn't heard from Shannon and Paul since they left the hospital and was desperate for updates about him. Indeed, there was a message, but it was just four sentences. Apparently, the Morells had slipped out of the hospital without any trouble. Shannon wrote that she was hoping to get her girls to preschool this week. The message had nothing about the baby.

Was this the way it was going to be?

I stared at the message for a while and then sent her a reply.

Glad to hear everything went smoothly for you. I hope you are able to get back to normal as soon as possible. Give Logan a kiss from us.

I could have told her I had been discharged, but I wasn't sure if she cared. I could have asked her questions about Logan, but I wasn't sure if she thought that was my business.

Does she care? Is Logan my business?

Maybe I wasn't thinking clearly, I thought. I was feverish and in pain, and I was completely exhausted. Some of this had to be hormones. I couldn't stop sobbing. My milk was coming in, and I had no baby to feed. I shook off the chilly message and went up to bed.

I knew I needed sleep, but when I shut my eyes and started to drift off, I found myself in a dark and stormy sea. I had fallen overboard, and I could barely stay afloat. Just out of reach in the turbulent waters, I could see my baby, but I couldn't get to him. He was sinking. I kicked and paddled desperately, but he disappeared under the water. I woke, panting and dripping with sweat. I was drowning. My baby was gone, and the terror was real. I felt like I had lost everything. That night I didn't even feel God. I was empty.

Perhaps this wasn't about Logan. Maybe it was about the baby that Jennifer was carrying for us. I felt like something was wrong with my baby. I tried to shrug it off, but I was tossing around. I didn't want to wake Sean. I went downstairs and checked my e-mail. There was another message from Shannon. This one was filled with details about Logan's first moments with his sisters and tidbits about how much he was adored by his grandparents. I was thankful for the message. Whatever possessed Shannon to e-mail me a second time that night I don't know, but thank goodness she did. I don't know what I would have done without that message.

Maybe you will get to be a part of his life.

After I read that message and knew Logan was well, I wondered about my dream and became convinced that something had happened to my baby. I thought of the ultrasound of our baby we received while I was in the hospital, and it occurred to me that I didn't know Jennifer was going for an appointment that day. I wondered if there was something wrong and no one wanted to tell me. I shot off an e-mail to her, asking if all was okay. The next morning she wrote back that the ultrasound was from a routine appointment and the baby looked great.

I hung on to the hope of our unborn child, and it kept me going as I tried to accept my new reality. I thought about Logan no less than I thought about Drew, Ryan, and MK. My new life included a perpetual state of wondering. What was Logan doing right then? Was he happy? Was he sick? Was he crying? Who was loving him this very moment? I didn't wonder about Drew, Ryan, and MK like this because I knew the answers to these questions. For a mother to have to wonder . . . constantly . . . is not a great way to live. I guess I knew he was alive, and that was a gift . . . unless he was being mistreated. I was spooking myself, because there was no reason to think that he was being anything but loved and adored.

At night before I fall asleep, I say my prayers and ask the angels to fly my love to my children. I've always imagined that my mom does the same for me—that her love comes to me at night and that it's the one thing that will always be. It helps me sleep too. When I got home from the hospital, I added Logan to my nightly prayer. I prayed that the angels would carry my love to Drew, Ryan, MK, and Logan. I imagined that when my love reached him, he was warmed by it and could relax into a peaceful sleep. That connection I felt to him from our time together was still strong for me. I genuinely felt like he was my baby.

Logan made me proud, gave me peace, caused me to grieve and to cry, sometimes all of it in the space of an hour. Buffeted between these strong bursts of feelings, I found it hard to navigate my way through the day. I hoped that the appointment I had scheduled at the end of the week with the counselor Dr. Read recommended could help me make sense of what I was feeling.

When I arrived at Linda Vanderpol's office, I was immediately comforted by her kind smile and complete understanding of the grief that was overwhelming me. Dr. Read had spoken with Linda since I made the appointment, so Linda knew the basics of my story. That meant that I couldn't fill up the time with the chronology of our last nine months and then skip out the door. I could sense how close to the surface all my emotions were, and I didn't want to parade them before a woman I barely knew. Yet all she had to do was ask a simple question and it all came tumbling out.

"How are you dealing with your feelings of loss?" she asked.

"Not well. It's not just the loss of Logan, it's the loss of our dreams for our family," I said. "I always thought I would be the 'mommy' and that my kids would grow up in my house, under my watchful eye, with my kisses being given to them every day. To know that there is a child out in the world that I gave life to, but he doesn't know me, is hard. Every grain in my being is saying that he is my baby and it's my job to protect him. I am his mother. My body gave him life but somehow didn't earn it. It breaks my heart to think about it. There were times when people referred to me as a surrogate for the Morell family. That sickens me. I wanted a baby for our family. But what I wanted and what I intended are suddenly meaningless."

"Do you feel isolated? Do you have friends you can lean on?"

"Oh, I have plenty of friends, and they are great women. The kind of friends who will be there for you no matter what," I said, thinking of my go-to friends JoAnn, Tracy, Linda, and Ann, and I also had the Reliable Girls. "But I think most people think it is over. The pregnancy is over, the baby is gone, and we should just get over it. Get our lives back. That will never happen."

"Do you dream about Logan?"

"Yes, I dream about him. I wonder about how he is doing. Does he miss me? Does he know that Shannon is not me?" I said. "You know, some people believe that children choose their parents. Did Logan choose us? What if he did, and we sent him away? What if he would have rather stayed with us in our family? I just don't know. I'll never know. So I granted compassion to Shannon and Paul, and at some level I still feel I'll never know if it was the right thing to do."

"So even though you feel connected to your husband and to your friends, you fear that no one can understand what you went through."

"Yes, no one can. Even Sean, who was right beside me. What I did is too odd, too unusual, and it's not even recognized in a court of law," I said. "I had no rights to the human being that was growing inside of me. He wasn't mine. I couldn't keep him. I could kill him, but I couldn't keep him. There is some serious irony in that. I meant nothing. I'm not sure I could have been made to feel more insignificant. I feel like nothing.

"I wonder if I will ever get over this? Will I think about this child for the rest of my life?" I pleaded. "I have wondered if when I die and my children are called, will they call him? Will he care? Will he understand what I did for him? Will he understand that I would do it all over again? I hope the sadness of giving him up will lessen someday, but I don't know how to stop this horrible movie that plays over and over again in my head."

"What movie?"

"The movie of Logan's birth. Him being taken out of my body, his first cry, his eyes opening and looking into my face, and the way he calmed when I spoke to him. When that part plays, I am so happy. But then comes the nightmare of the nurses taking him away. The terror of that moment cripples me." I started to cry. "I hope someday I don't feel so empty. I'm not sure that will happen, though. I think that I will just somehow be able to weave the sadness into the fabric of my life and continue to focus on the positive. That's what I want to do. That's what I want help to do. I want to enjoy life as I did before. I don't want to cheat my family out of my happiness."

"Carolyn, I know you came here for postpartum depression," the counselor said. "But you have post-traumatic stress disorder."

Post-traumatic stress disorder? I thought PTSD was a diagnosis re-

served for military veterans, survivors of horrific accidents, or vic-
tims of heinous crimes. What we had been through in the last eight
months was soul-shaking, but did PTSD describe me? I knew that it
was a serious diagnosis, one that wouldn't be cured with a prescription and a few trips to a therapist.

"Are you sure that is what I have?"

"I have no doubt," she said. "This is going to take a long while
to heal. You have to be patient with yourself, compassionate, and
I think you could use some antidepressants to keep some of your
darker feelings at bay."

I had never been on antidepressants before, but was aware that it
was a treatment that could really help my mood. Still, I had always
been confident that I'd never suffer from depression. Linda helped
me understand that there was no way that a person gets through life
without experiencing at least a mild depression at some point.

"It's nothing to be ashamed of. You see, Carolyn, you have not
only lived through a horrific loss, you have endured eight months
in which you were continually tortured," she said. "I wish I would
have seen you sooner. In order to recover, you're going to need to
cut yourself some slack, take this medication, continue in therapy,
and work hard toward becoming whole again."

I hadn't really thought of my pregnancy as torture, but I appreciated the comparison. I knew that we had suffered profoundly and
that I was continuously replaying in my head the moment of Logan's
birth, followed by the moment when they took him away from me.
We had talked about our suffering many times with Kevin Anderson,
but we'd always assumed that the suffering would diminish after the
delivery. Now I was sure that we were going to suffer for a long time.

Eight days after Logan was born, Sean's sister Patti brought me
lunch. My mom had left that morning, and I appreciated Patti's
company that afternoon. As we were sitting in the family room
chatting, my home phone rang. I checked the caller ID, recognized
an out-of-state area code, and decided not to answer, thinking it was

more media. The ringing stopped, but a minute later my cell phone rang. When I glanced at that caller ID, I saw the same number.

It couldn't be the media. They didn't have my cell phone number.

"Hello?" I said quietly, afraid that I shouldn't have been answering. When there was no reply, I almost hung up, but could hear the cries of a woman through the receiver. It was then that I recognized the area code as Indianapolis.

"Jennifer?"

"Carolyn?" was all Jennifer could manage between her sobs.

"Jennifer? Oh, my God, what's wrong? Are you okay?" Jennifer was struggling to speak.

"Carolyn, they couldn't find a heartbeat."

"What?"

"I'm so sorry. We double-checked. They sent me to the hospital, but there was no heartbeat."

"Jennifer, are you alone? Are you driving?"

She could barely talk, and I was scared that she was trying to drive while talking to me on her cell.

"Pull over. It's okay. We've been through this before. It's not your fault."

"I'm sorry. I'm so sorry."

I could only imagine how scared she was to make this phone call. She knew we had only said good-bye to Logan a week before.

"It's not your fault. This has happened to us before. You need to calm down."

I could hear her breathing slowing, and I was surprising myself with the calm manner in which I was reacting.

"You'll need a D&C. We'll take care of that. We'll take care of everything. Please don't worry. We don't blame you. This kind of thing happens. We'll be okay."

I could hear the words leaving my mouth.

We'll be okay? We would? We only lost Logan last week. Now this? Seriously?

Patti was sitting on my couch, staring at me with her mouth hanging open. We were waiting until we had safely cleared the first trimester to tell people Jennifer was carrying our baby. By hearing my end of the conversation, Patti had inferred what happened. Having miscarried twice herself, she understood the loss.

"I'm so sorry. What do you want me to do?" Patti asked.

What could she do? What could anyone do?

"I need to call Sean," I said. I took the phone in the other room and dialed his cell number. He answered immediately.

"Jennifer miscarried," I mumbled as I huddled on a chair in the corner of our home office.

"I am so sorry. I am on my way home," he said.

I hung up the phone, numb.

I couldn't believe how I couldn't manage any tears. Were my tears all used up?

The best way out is through. I remembered Kevin Anderson's words.

But I thought I was through. How much more was there?

I wasn't sure I wanted the answer to that question. I pulled my legs to my chest and dropped my face into the dark hollow between my knees and my chest. I had nothing left. No more tears, no more grief, and no more room for greater loss. I stared out the window and listened to Patti playing with Mary Kate in the family room.

You have to get up, go back in there, explain what happened, and move on. You have to move on for your kids. For Sean.

I would trudge onward, with an empty heart, and pray for someone to point me to the best way out.

SEAN

I WALKED THROUGH the door and Patti left to give us some time. As I approached Carolyn I broke down as we embraced. I hugged her tight to my chest, trying to give her comfort, but also because I needed comfort.

I spoke first. "Why, why this now? I feel like a boxer who was knocked down, gathered himself while leaning on the ropes, and then a body blow comes and finishes him off."

"Sean, I know. There is nothing left to cry out."

This miscarriage hurt more than the others, even though Carolyn wouldn't suffer the physical effects. We were so tapped out by the loss of Logan that I didn't think we had room for any more sorrow. This was the one hope we'd held on to for most of the pregnancy with Logan. As we embraced we were holding each other up. I do not believe either of us could have stood alone. Two blows in eight days.

As with the pregnancy, Carolyn and I worked hard in the days after Jennifer's miscarriage to keep the boys' schedules intact. The news of the miscarriage came just a week before the championship that was the culmination of Ryan's cross-country season. Although it pained me to leave Carolyn, we agreed that I should fulfill my commitment to coach Ryan and the whole team at the meet. Ryan was having a great season and was becoming a real leader for the younger runners to emulate.

The night before the championship, my sleep was restless. I woke at 5:00 A.M. with a hollow feeling in the pit of my stomach. I looked at Carolyn sleeping and knew that her emptiness was tremendous. I didn't want to leave her. *I need to get through this day. My son needs me to be there. My team needs me to be there, and I need me to be there.*

I slipped on my clothes for my morning run, which usually wakes me up and helps me focus before the meet. Alone with my thoughts, I reflected on my friend Mike joining me for a long run this past week as a sign of support, and my friend Dan checking in on me yesterday just to see if there was anything he could do. This outside support helped, but my internal sadness was ever present. Three miles of running in the crsip fall air did little to help. I was torn between wanting to embrace the day and wanting to hide. I needed to embrace the day. Carolyn said that she was going to rally enough to come watch Ryan, so I had to do my part too.

I arrived at the meet about 6:30 and dragged the tents and tarp and table to our regular spot to set up. The sun was just making its way above the horizon, and since no one from our team would arrive for a while, I went for a walk to gather my thoughts. Out of view of anyone, I sat on the ground with my face in my hands. I could not keep from thinking about what we'd been through. My mind then moved to a memory of Carolyn and me holding each other just after we heard about the miscarriage. She was barely functioning. Being alone was not a good idea for either of us right now. Bad images flooded my brain. *Why me? Why us? Why now?* I was feeling sorry for myself. *Just stand up and walk back. This day needs your attention. Everyone has worked so hard to get to this point, and you need to be a leader and not wallow in self-pity.*

I returned to the tent and found that my fellow coach and close friend Steve Baugh had arrived to set up. "Sean, is this the day?" Steve asked when I returned to our table. I knew what he was referring to, but I pretended not to hear him. No team had ever won all eight divisions of the CYO cross-country championships in the thirty-five-year history of the event. Our team of 160 runners had trained hard and put in consistent performances. Steve and I had often talked about wanting to be the first school to finish first in every division.

"Sean, is this the year?"

"We've got a chance," I said, worrying about jinxing the day.

Ryan and his teammates performed tremendously on a brilliant day, scoring success after success. At the end of the meet, we had eight first-place trophies stacked up on our table in the tent next to my cross-country binder. There was incredible excitement around the tent as all the kids celebrated their great success. Twenty-four parent volunteer coaches were also all smiles. Steve and I approached each other and said simultaneously, "We did it!"

As I was walking toward my car to leave, one of the younger runners yelled, "Coach! Coach!"

I turned and leaned down to get close to Jimmy.

"Coach, what the team did today, we did it for you."

A chill went down my spine as I smiled, not thinking about the first-place finishes but thinking more about the love. Everyone knew what Carolyn and I had been going through. During all those lonely days, we had never really been abandoned, even though it felt like it sometimes. We had been in everyone's thoughts and prayers. Logan was born, and that phase of our crisis was complete. Now I could really sense the love of my community.

That evening we closed the cross-country season with our traditional banquet, attended by about four hundred people. I opened by saying thank you to the team, to the coaches, to the parents, " . . . and to my wife."

I scanned the crowd and caught her eyes.

"Carolyn, I thank you for allowing me the time and providing me with the support to keep coaching this. . . ." As I looked out at the crowd, I saw a lot of tears. I could not finish my statement. I broke down and despite my efforts could not continue.

I left that evening thankful for the St. Joe's community and for Carolyn. She had always been there supporting me with my career, my coaching, and so many other projects I jumped into over the past twenty-one years. As I looked out in the crowd to thank her, I was overcome with a sense of admiration and love for what she had been through. I will never know what it was like to walk in her shoes the past eight months, and all I can do is walk beside her as we move forward together.

CHAPTER 22

Ambiguous Loss

SEAN

As we walked into Kevin's office for our first appointment after the delivery, we were struggling with loss. Even with the eight months we'd had to prepare ourselves to hand Logan to the Morells, our brief time with him face to face had left an immeasurable void. Compounding the loss of Logan, we were now dealing with the miscarriage of our own child. Not only was the grief overwhelming, but we also had a kind of yearning that I'd never experienced.

Sometimes it was a sweet yearning filled with love for the new baby. Other times it was a desperate, almost angry yearning, knowing that we had been so close to him and now he was gone at the same moment when our sliver of a hope for a child with Jennifer vanished too. Of course, we remained resigned to the fact—and even took pride in it—that we had decided not to mount a custody battle. Paul and Shannon were Logan's rightful parents, and we hoped and believed they would be very good and devoted parents. But the heart does not know logic. Carolyn and I felt like we were his parents the whole time he was nurtured by her womb, and we were also the parents of the baby who died in the miscarriage. Those are primal bonds, a kind of fierce connection to an unborn child that is vital for a man who is sacrificing to protect the family.

Those feelings were deep in our blood, and our child was gone, but not gone.

I kept to my routine. I went to work early, as I always had, and fulfilled my responsibilities to my family, but our loss seemed to be on every surface that I touched, on every street corner I passed. I never knew that the absence of something could become immense. The loss of Logan and the miscarriage muted my senses. I was dulled by these losses, and try as I might, I couldn't shake the feeling that our lives had become grayer and might be that way for some time.

As the session started, I decided to share first and to focus on Logan. My images of that day were still so strong in my mind.

"Kevin, the birth was beautiful, and there was tremendous satisfaction in delivering Logan to Paul and Shannon. Then, after they left the hospital, we were stricken with grief. I have a difficult time describing the loss. Is it grief we are feeling? Or something else?"

"You are dealing with ambiguous loss," he said. "A loss of something that is not really gone, like when a child is abducted. The child is physically gone, but the psychological attachment of the parents is still there. They grieve this person even though they hope and pray that he or she is still alive. They can feel the loss constantly. Many children feel ambiguous loss when their parents divorce. Your loss is so much different than that, though. The baby is elsewhere, presumably happy and well. He is alive in your minds and in your hearts, but you can't see or touch him. Sean and Carolyn, the grief of a loss like this may fade over time, but ambiguous loss never goes away. Your grief seems frozen in place."

"Frozen" was a good word for what I was feeling.

"Every day we deal with the loss of Logan," I said. "Carolyn has the physical reminders daily of the pregnancy and her body seeking to nourish the child. I have nightmares of someone trying to break into our home to take our other children. This is all-consuming."

"There's no ritual for this loss," Carolyn said. "It would be wrong to have a funeral or a baby shower. A year from now, we

won't exactly be having a birthday party for him or a one-year anniversary for his passing out of our lives. We have no public way to
honor the significance of his passing, so we can't find a way to shut
the door. And we don't want to walk away. We love him."

"Logan did not die on September 24, but he died to us as parents," I said. "I will not be his father. I will not be able to hold him
in my arms or coach him on the cross-country or on the basketball
team or play catch with him in the backyard. To him, I will be no
different than any other person on the street. As he grows I expect
I'll continue to think about what I would be doing with him at that
particular stage of life. Every time I think of Logan like that, I'll
feel this loss."

"Are you familiar with Kahlil Gibran's poem 'On Children'?"
Kevin asked.

We shook our heads.

"In *The Prophet*, he writes:

> *Your children are not your children.*
> *They are the sons and daughters of Life's longing for itself.*
> *They come through you but not from you,*
> *And though they are with you yet they belong not to you.*

Carolyn and I looked at each other with a flash of mutual recog-
nition. This was the kind of sentiment that hit you in the heart first.
The logical mind took a few more seconds to get it.

"But it's human nature to lay claim to our children almost as if
they are a possession. I do it with my kids. Who are they if they are
not our own?" I asked.

"Gibran would say that parents bring life into the world," Kevin
said. "Life's longing to continue is manifest in the love and opti-
mism of that act and in the daily attentions you pay to your children. But they are not really yours. They belong to the world. They
belong to their own lives and to their destinies."

"Carolyn and I having children is our contribution to life's continuation," I said, trying to express it in my own way. "Children are a gift from God, and children entering this world through us is not a continuation of us. Our time here is finite."

"Yes, it is," Kevin said. "Consider what you did for Logan in this light."

Yes, we did this for Logan. In the beginning, we did it because we were people who wanted to be true to our values. As the pregnancy progressed and we fell in love with the baby Carolyn carried, our focus changed. We were doing this because we loved this child and we wished him the best life possible. Whether we were part of that life was something we couldn't and shouldn't cling to.

"Logan is the son of Life's longing for itself in the truest sense," I said. "We gave Logan life, and then we had to let him go. We had to release him completely, not knowing if he will ever come back. The loss is so powerful, but we take comfort in allowing Logan to make his way in this world and live out his destiny."

"Exactly. This is a gift," Kevin said. His eyes were grave and his manner was somber. "You gave a tremendous gift to the Morells. When you give a gift, you are not depleted by that generosity. It is a sign of the best aspects of who you are."

I shut my eyes. Yes, Logan was a gift to the Morells, and I was proud of how we had handled his birth. But there was no denying how much both of us were hurting.

"Children are a gift from God," I said with conviction. "Children are our gift to the world. Those who hold too tightly to their children will drive them away and be left broken-hearted," I said. "Children need to be given independence. I believe children come from us with God's grace and that we as parents have tremendous influence over their character and development, but that they need to be given freedom to make their own choices and find their place in this world."

I thought of Drew, Ryan, and Mary Kate. Every day we had

with them they were slowly gaining independence. We were their protectors and their role models, but with every decision they made on their own they moved toward that separation. Over the course of the decades they lived with us, we could gradually let go. Logan had been with us for mere minutes.

As Carolyn and I left the session I was so thankful that we had welcomed Kevin into our lives. Not because he soothed away my grief. He didn't. This loss was everywhere I looked, but Kevin's counsel had opened this loss to the world. I felt it in my heart, but I could also feel some connection to the millions of other parents who have lost a child, holding that baby for only a brief moment or never having that opportunity before he was gone. So many people suffer devastating losses, and it seemed wrong to compare what Carolyn and I were going through to anyone else. Each is powerful in its own right. Instead, I felt connected to those experiencing loss, whatever it might be. Tapping into this well of grief from so many helped dissipate its power over me. I could pour this inexhaustible grief up into the sky. Kevin helped me see that our grief might never completely leave and that closure will not come. That did not mean there is no room for hope. Instead of seeking closure, we needed to turn our focus to a search for meaning. The search would take time, maybe a lifetime, but I believed it begins with sharing our experience in an effort to help others. The Jesuits believe the way to live is to become a "man for others," and that is a worthy endeavor. If Carolyn and I can be of help to others, then in return we will be helped and meaning will be revealed.

CAROLYN

ONLY A FEW PEOPLE knew we had a miscarriage, and I had never been so grateful in my life that I had kept my mouth shut about something. We didn't have to make anyone feel any worse for us than they already did. Our family and friends already didn't know what to say to us. How would they even find the most rudimentary words to soothe us about another loss?

Jennifer had a dilation and curettage to remove what was left of her pregnancy ten days after Logan was born, and thankfully, she came through the surgery without complications. We had genetic testing done on the fetus in hopes of learning a cause, but regardless of what those results might tell us, the sting of our loss was tearing at our hearts. Later I learned that our baby had stopped developing the day I came home from the hospital, the night of my dream. Was it my baby that was drowning in the water?

You were connected to your child. You knew.

Things were pretty bleak, but one thing that kept our spirits lifted was the mail from well-wishers from around the world. There were so many letters that our mailman was bringing the mail to our door in tubs. Every night Sean and I would sift through letters from strangers who had been touched by what we did for Logan.

Dear Sean and Carolyn,

I'm just a granny from South Carolina, and I wanted to thank you for saving that babe. I can assure you, his granny is even more thankful than I am. God bless.

Dear Mr. and Mrs. Savage,

I can only imagine the sadness you are feeling right now. Please know, that your story has touched me in a way that I cannot express. Thank you for your courage, and restoring faith in the power of the human spirit and the capacity for kindness. May your tribe increase.

Some envelopes were addressed simply "Sean and Carolyn Savage, the Mixed Up Embryo Couple," but the U.S. Postal Service got it enough to get these messages of love and comfort to us. Every night when Sean came home from work, he marveled at the heap of letters strewn across the kitchen table. Drew and Ryan, who kept track of the arrivals, said that we had heard from someone in about every state in the country. Interestingly, many of the writers said that they had never been compelled to write to a stranger before but we had inspired them to reach out. Thank goodness they did, because those bright sentiments saw us through the darkness of our days.

In addition to hearing from strangers, there was one day about a month after Logan's birth when I received two packages. I carried them from the front porch to my kitchen, then opened the smaller one first.

"What is it, Mom?" Ryan was hoping it was candy.

"It's not anything to eat. I'm sure it is something about Logan," I said. I removed the treasure from the box and unfolded the tissue that surrounded it.

"What is it?"

It was from my friend Anne, who years ago lost a baby to a cord accident when she was thirty-nine weeks pregnant. We had talked about her baby, John, many times during my pregnancy. She had been a great adviser and helped prepare me for Logan's loss.

"It's from a friend" was all I said.

I smiled at Ryan, told him I needed a moment, and carried the gift into my office and shut the door.

Once I had some privacy, I picked up the package and stared at the silver picture frame engraved with the date of Logan's birth. *September 24, 2009.* Anne understood that the moment of Logan's birth was a moment to be treasured forever. I went to the pile of pictures we had snapped in the hospital and chose one of our entire family. For one glorious hour, on September 25, I had all of my babies together, and now I had a place to honor that moment. It was perfect.

"Mom!" Ryan yelled. "Are you going to open the next present?"

This one was larger, and I recognized the sender as one of my sorority sisters, Beth, from my years at Miami University.

Styrofoam peanuts fell all over the counter as I lifted out another box that had been decorated by one of Beth's kids and labeled "Carolyn's Sunshine Box." Inside were heaps of fun trinkets and pick-me-ups, a spa gift certificate, and. . .

"Yes! Chocolate!" Ryan said as he snatched the box of Godiva chocolates and ran to the family room. I chased him as I wrestled the box from him.

"I'll share, child, but one thing you need to learn: never snatch chocolate from a hormonal woman. It is dangerous."

After rationing Ryan a few pieces, I went back to the Sunshine Box and found a card. Apparently Beth had reached out via Facebook to over fifty sorority sisters of mine. Most of these women I hadn't heard from in almost twenty years. The idea that they cared so much about me now, after all this time, overwhelmed me, and before I knew it I was curled up on my chair, in my office, with my Kleenex and what was left of the chocolates trying to pull myself together.

The truth was that I felt gutted, but stuffing that empty space with chocolate after chocolate wouldn't fill it. The previous day, when I had been making salad for dinner, I stood over the sink with a cucumber in my hand. Standing up for long periods of time still caused me to ache, so I had to steady my forearms on the edge of the sink. I peeled the cucumber and sliced it in half lengthwise. With half of it in my left hand, I gutted it, scraping a spoon gently along the inside and loosening the seeds so they fell into the sink. When I picked up the other half, it hit me that that was exactly how I felt. I felt as though someone had scooped out my insides and thrown them in the trash. That image was so powerful to me that I shared it with Linda at my next appointment.

"What do you think it will take to feel like you haven't been gutted?"

"I actually don't know if I will ever feel like I wasn't gutted.

I guess I'll just learn to live with the feeling. Like it is part of me. I don't think it will ever go away. There is a hole inside of me. A missing part. Logan is the missing part, and now I realize that there is not a circumstance in the world that will ever bring him back to me. Nothing."

"Would a new baby make you feel better?"

"No. I could have more babies, but they won't replace him. I'll always feel like something is missing. I guess the part of me that is missing left with him."

"That is grief. You know that, right?"

"I understand."

I did understand. He was just gone from our lives, and no one could tell me how long it would take for me to recover. No one had an answer.

CHAPTER 23

Godspeed

CAROLYN

EVEN THOUGH OUR HEARTS were wounded, Sean and I got out of bed every morning to tackle the day. There was some solace in that. Kevin said that people who suffer ambiguous loss are frozen in grief. But the world was moving on, and we needed to move with it. Nothing provided complete relief from my sorrow, though. I worried constantly about Logan. I knew that he was in Shannon's capable hands, but didn't he need me? If he needed me, I should be there. If he didn't need me, that hurt too. One time I was on the phone with Shannon, and I heard a cry in the background and wondered, *Is that him? Is that a hungry cry? Is that a sleepy cry? Is that a diaper change cry?*

I thought back to the days when I first brought my babies home and started trying to figure out what made them cry or what soothed them. I wondered what Logan was like in the morning. Was he a sunny little soul like MK? Or was he a cranky pants like Ryan, whose best hours were always in the afternoon?

I hesitated to ask Shannon for details. I didn't want to intrude. Yet anytime my mind touched on Logan's name, my image was of him resting on my chest at the hospital or the moment of bliss when I heard his first cry. I had no other image to add to that. When Shannon had told me that she had professional photos taken of Logan in October, I'd asked her to please send me a copy, and I'd picked out a frame to put it in. I'd even started an album for Logan, but I hadn't had anything to put in it since he left the hospital.

I checked my e-mail way too often, hoping always for a message from Shannon. I thought of pathetic reasons to reach out when I was desperate for some news. Once I e-mailed Shannon asking for toy recommendations for Mary Kate. Even a discussion about plastic versus wooden toy kitchens made me feel as though the connection between Logan and me was alive.

I longed for a newborn to cuddle, and I called the clinic in Atlanta to check on the last two embryos we'd stored there.

"You're going to think I'm nuts, but I have to be sure," I said. "Are my embryos really there?"

The nurse paused before answering my question.

"Of course they're here," she said. "They are in a straw in the tank in our lab."

"Have you seen them? Can you check? Are you sure they are labeled correctly?" I asked. "I know this sounds crazy."

"They are safe, Mrs. Savage," the nurse said. "When we heard what happened to you and your family, we checked and double-checked our protocols for everyone."

These were our last remaining embryos—our last chance, as we thought of them. Jennifer felt so bad about the miscarriage and was almost as eager as we were to try one more time. After I reconfirmed with the clinic our plan to move forward with a final transfer in January, I hung up and sat for a while in the study.

Carolyn, you must focus on the blessings in front of you.

Drew was nearing the end of his cross-country season, and Sean was working and coaching Ryan's basketball team. MK and I were very busy too. I paused to thank God for my family. I felt grateful for how much was already in my life.

Even after I admonished myself to move on, I stayed somewhat stuck.

"It's been two weeks since we heard anything," I told Sean one night when he got home from work.

"Is Shannon back to work?"

"I don't think so. Last I heard she was extending her leave until after Thanksgiving," I said. "Don't you wonder what color his eyes are?"

"Aren't they blue? Paul and Shannon both have blue eyes. I think that means his will be blue too."

"I wonder what shade of blue they are."

"Haven't we gotten a picture?"

"Not since September. I hope we'll get a Christmas card or something."

"Can we ask for one?"

"I don't know. I don't want to overstep."

One afternoon in November I was driving the kids back from school when I stopped to collect the mail from our box. Mixed in with the bills and holiday catalogs was a royal blue envelope with the Morells' return address.

"Finally! A picture of my Little Man!"

The envelope was stiff in my hand. I ripped it open and flung the envelope to the floor of the car.

"No, it's a card. A card with a picture?"

The front of the card featured an adorable picture of the entire Morell family. I squinted at the tiny baby curled up in the middle. I could barely see his face. The caption read:

A New Baby is the Beginning of All Things.
Wonder, Hope & A Dream of Possibilities.

"Is this a birth announcement?"

Inside the card was a picture of him captioned.

Logan Savage Morell. . .
9–24–09 . . . 5 lbs 3oz . . . 18 inches. . .
Welcomed Home with Love
Paul, Shannon, Ellie and Megan.

I couldn't look at it. I dropped the card to my lap and drove to our house. Drew got out of the car and grabbed his gear from the back of the van.

"Aren't you coming, Mom?"

"I just need to read this. I'll be right in."

As the door to the house shut behind him, I looked down at the birth announcement.

This is good, Carolyn. They are celebrating Logan's birth and their blessings. This is good!

Good? How was this good? This should have been our announcement. We should have been the happy family with the fruits of my labor curled up on my lap. I looked at my lap. My C-section wasn't healed. Dr. Read's estimate of when my milk would dry up was wrong. I was still leaking.

Get over it, Carolyn. He is not yours. This is the way it's going to be.

I wiped my tears with my sleeve and got out of the car. Dinner had to be made, homework needed to be done, and MK needed a bath.

Onward, Carolyn. Onward.

That night in the rocking chair, when I read to Mary Kate, I asked myself where God was in this. If God was everywhere and in everything, was he in that birth announcement that had stung me so? Every day since February 16, 2009, I had muttered a futile prayer. *Please help me.* Sometimes I had begged for God's help with my head buried in the loo with morning sickness, or at night when reflux woke me, or when Logan wouldn't stop kicking. Other times that plea had come to me as I drove home from a prenatal appointment in anguish over our inevitable loss. When I felt no relief, when the agony persisted, I'd asked myself: *Who am I praying to? Who am I begging? Why won't God help me?*

I know He exists. I've felt his powerful and unmistakable presence three times in my life. The first time was when I was in the hospital recovering from pneumonia the week Ryan was born. My cough was relentless, and when I asked the nurse for a cough drop, she suggested that I buy some Lifesavers from the vending machines. I dragged myself into the hallway and shuffled toward the vending machines dragging my IV pole. Sean had gone home for the night, so I was on my own, and the vending machines seemed like they were a very long way away. I didn't think I had the strength to get there.

You'll be fine.

I heard a voice and felt a firm hand on my back. I trudged steadily, that hand guiding me around the corner, into the waiting room, and to the machines. I retrieved the Lifesavers and found my way to my room, grateful that my companion was right by my side. Back in my room, I turned to thank the nurse and then realized no one was there. Had someone been with me?

You didn't do that alone.

Eleven years later, I lay in a hospital bed twenty-four hours after the birth of Mary Kate. My red blood cell count was dangerously low, and I'd had a terrible reaction to magnesium sulfate, the only medication that was controlling my alarmingly high blood pressure. Yet I felt that there was someone holding me safely as my bed seemed to spin around the room. He rubbed my head when a fierce headache stabbed me right between my eyes. I could see Him.

I was there.

I've realized that during each of these experiences I was in an altered state, and I used to wonder if maybe I needed to be in that state to open my senses to His presence. Either way, now I no longer doubted that He was with me. Why I couldn't always see God's presence was a question I couldn't answer. Was He trying to show me that He is always there, always close at hand, but that He only reveals Himself when I'm at my most vulnerable?

I didn't know the answer to that question until last February, when I saw Him the third time. That afternoon, as I lay in bed waiting for the results of my pregnancy test, God revealed Himself to me again. I was sick and weak with a fever and chills, and I'd drifted off to sleep with my phones on my pillow, waiting for the clinic to confirm that I was pregnant. As I dozed off, I felt Him near, but I was confused.

"Why are you here?" I asked. "I'm not sick like the other times."

There was no answer.

"I don't need you. I am okay with however this goes. Why are you here?"

Nothing but silence.

I woke knowing something wasn't right. Then I heard Sean coming up the stairs to our bedroom, the door opened, and our journey began.

There were countless times during my pregnancy when I felt abandoned. I wanted to be sheltered and cared for. Despite my weaknesses and doubts, God was there. Now I realize that He revealed Himself to me in that moment because He knew I was headed for a potential spiritual disaster. If I didn't maintain my faith, I would lose myself in sorrow. Even though I couldn't always see Him or feel Him, He walked my path with me. The night we learned of the mistake, I couldn't imagine surviving this heartbreak and coming out the other side okay. On that day, when it all began, He was reminding me not to lose faith.

He guided me to do the right thing. But now I needed God more than ever as I struggled to let Logan go.

Shannon had sent me a birth announcement for Logan at the same time and in the same way that she had announced him to her extended family and distant friends. This was what stabbed at my soul. I was now a bystander in his life.

When I got back downstairs, I looked at the picture of Logan in the birth announcement. He wore the outfit I had tucked into the treasure chest for him. His feet were perfect, and his fingers were long. He was too young to smile, but he was surrounded by the happy faces of his family. This was an announcement that my job was done. I had to let Logan go and try to find a way to feel good about that. I saw Logan in this beautiful picture. He was healthy, well cared for, and clearly adored by his parents. Who was to say I could love him any better than they did?

I had to accept the reality of this situation. This was things as they were, and I could not hope for more. Carefully I cut the picture from the birth announcement and placed it in the frame I'd bought.

God, I feel you now. I feel your eyes on me. I have done your will. Please be merciful and grant me peace.

SEAN

NO STRINGS ATTACHED. That was our approach to giving Logan to Paul and Shannon. I believe that a gift with conditions is not a gift at all. Throughout the pregnancy, we consistently communicated to Paul and Shannon that we would defer to them on deciding when we could see Logan. That just made sense to us. I couldn't picture calling the Morells and announcing, "I will be at your home next Saturday to spend time with your son." We waited to be invited when they felt it was right. Carolyn and I believed it was the proper approach. Paul and Shannon needed to determine what was best for their family. There was no road map for either of us, so Carolyn and I challenged ourselves to find compassion for Paul and Shannon in their struggle to find the best way to handle this moving forward.

On my first day back at work after the birth, my assistant Laura wanted to know when I thought I would see Logan again.

"I don't know," I said. "We're happy to see him whenever they will let us. We need to leave it up to them."

"I'm sure you'll see him soon," said Laura brightly.

Little did I know that many people would ask that same question.

Nearly every client I met with wanted to know, and so did everyone I bumped into at the office kitchen. Before Logan was born, people often asked if we would really want to see the baby once we had handed him over to the other family. I understood that they wanted to protect us and believed that seeing him would be a painful reminder of our loss. I think what other people really wanted to ask was, "Don't you want to forget this ever happened?" How could we pretend this did not happen? Why would we really want to do that? A beautiful child was involved, and this had been a life-changing process.

As the days turned to weeks and then to months without seeing Logan, I often looked at the photograph of our time with him in the hospital. Carolyn had placed it in a silver frame in our living room. We are all frozen in that moment when Carolyn, myself, Drew, Ryan, and Mary Kate bonded with Logan. Relaxed, happy, and excited were the emotions running through me in that picture. The "family" picture taken during that visit will be the only one of its kind. Logan will grow and change, but our most powerful image will be the baby we held in our hands on September 25, 2009.

I envisioned ten years down the road, driving to a ball field and parking my car in a spot where I could watch Logan play from a distance. Maybe I would catch him smiling, or interacting with his friends, or walking away from the game with his parents describing a play he'd made, or crying about a tough loss. The other image I have is of Carolyn and me sneaking into a church on Logan's wedding day to watch with pride as he gets married. I see us doing these things in a manner that draws no attention to us but honors our love for him. Seeing him in person participating in his life would be a thrill. There would be satisfaction in those moments, a satisfaction that Carolyn and I would share and treasure.

I hoped that time and reflection would give me perspective on this. Carolyn and I had no idea how our relationship with Logan would unfold or how it was supposed to unfold. I drew inspiration from a picture I once saw of Mother Teresa in an orphanage in which she has her arms stretched to welcome the children. I was confident that Carolyn and I would always be ready, with our arms open, to welcome Logan at any time we were blessed with a visit.

I have one other vision I treasure that comes to me when I think of Logan's future and our relationship with him. I have imagined a day eighteen years from now when we hear a knock on the door. We answer, and a handsome young man stands in front of us and simply says, "Thank you for giving me life." If he grows up with gratitude in his heart, we could ask for nothing more. Godspeed, Logan.

CAROLYN

BY THE TIME THANKSGIVING rolled around and we still had no firm plans to see Logan, Sean started joking about showing up at the Morells' house with a turkey. Needless to say, I didn't think this was such good idea. As Christmas neared, I was beginning to wonder if we'd ever see him. Shortly before Christmas, we finally set a date. The Morells would bring their whole family to visit on December 29, just about three months after he was born.

It was a sunny day, and the landscape of northwest Ohio was blanketed with snow. I ran around making sure everything was perfect. I cleaned the playroom, dusted off some of MK's old baby toys, and straightened our tired and very dry Christmas tree.

As I rearranged ornaments that had fallen from the brittle branches, I came across the impression of Logan's foot that our nurse had made for us in the delivery room and moved it to a more prominent place on the tree. I wondered how big his feet were now.

The Morells were supposed to arrive at 3:00 P.M., but they were running a little late. It was nerve-racking for Sean and me to wait for Logan's arrival. By 3:15, Sean was peering out our bedroom window with the excitement of a child awaiting the arrival of Santa Claus. Three-thirty came and went, and then 3:45 and 4:00.

At 4:00 Sean decided to change his luck and went downstairs to look out different windows. Soon he was pacing the family room, worrying that they'd been in a car accident or had decided not to come. I was perched on the couch in the living room, staring out the window for the first sign of Shannon's van. We couldn't even be in the same room. Like Sean, I was nervous to see my Little Man. I was afraid of falling apart. *You won't do that.* I was frightened that he wouldn't come to me. *He's not old enough to have a fear of strangers.* I was petrified that the Morells wouldn't show. *They'd never do that.* I knew they were getting closer. *Could I feel him?*

"They're here! They're here!" Sean yelled and sprinted to my side.

I saw Shannon's car come around the curve of our road and creep down our street until they made the turn into our driveway.

"You okay?" Sean said.

"I'm fine. I'll be cool. No worries," I said.

When I opened the door, I saw Paul holding the most beautiful baby boy, bundled head to toe under a blanket in his car seat. Paul came in and placed the carrier on the kitchen counter as Shannon guided the twins into our home. Paul uncovered Logan and pulled his hat off. My Little Man had huge chunky cheeks, a belly that looked well fed, and the most beautiful eyes I had ever seen on a baby.

His eyes are crystal clear blue!

I had an answer.

I didn't want to look too desperate. I understood that this couldn't be comfortable for Paul and Shannon. I followed Shannon into the family room, and we all sat down while Paul remained behind to change Logan's diaper. We made chitchat about the drive, until Paul walked in holding Logan. He came right to me with his son. I stood up and reached out, and without any hesitation, Paul placed Logan right into my arms.

If I could have stopped time, I would have. I wrapped my arms around Logan's chubby little body and instinctively pulled him to my chest. I imagined a puzzle piece snapping into place in that moment. As though the rest of my lungs had just been inflated. His head instinctively tucked in under my chin, and I lowered my face and kissed him gently on his head.

"Hi, sweetie," I said. I caught Sean's eye. He was watching me carefully, but with love and pride. Later he said I looked as though I was trying to download every feature of Logan's face to update my brain files. I smiled back. We were reading one another's minds.

Sean and I handed him off to one another, politely fighting over who was getting a fair "turn" at snuggling with the baby. The twins played with MK. Drew and Ryan both took turns doting over Logan. At one moment, Mary Kate walked by, smiled at Logan, and murmured "baby"—a far different response than she'd had in September. We'd all grown a little.

At one point, Logan needed a new diaper, and I offered to change him. I took him back to the changing table in our laundry room, and Sean followed me as if he was coming to help. I laid Logan down, and he looked up and smiled and cooed.

"What a happy child."

"You want to make a run for it?" Sean quipped.

I laughed, shook my head, picked Logan up, and walked back into the family room and handed him to Shannon for his bottle.

As she fed him, I watched. She was fastidious with him. The burp cloth was tucked under his chin to prevent formula dribble, which I knew would make my mom happy. He was clearly adored by his mommy and daddy, and he was dressed to the nines in a pair of brown corduroy overalls and matching socks, which I loved.

When I noticed his feet, I looked to his footprint that hung on our tree.

He is growing.

Shannon cuddled him to her while he ate, and then he settled in on her shoulder for a snooze.

He fits with her. He belongs to her.

Before I knew it, it was approaching nine o'clock, time for them to go. We all said our good-byes, and Sean and I thanked them again and again for bringing Logan for this visit. I watched Paul strap Logan into his car seat. Once again, he placed Logan on the counter. He asked me to watch Logan while they loaded the twins into the car. I stuck my face in the seat and got nose to nose with my Little Man.

"Bye-bye, sweetie. Mama loves you. Don't ever forget that. Know that in your heart, Little Man." I kissed him gently on the forehead.

Paul came back in to carry Logan to the car. As I watched them pull out of the driveway and off into the darkness, I surprised myself. I wasn't overcome with grief. I felt more of a relief from the emptiness in my heart.

I lay in bed that night with a feeling of gratitude that I hadn't felt before. Not only was I grateful to Paul and Shannon for allowing us a visit, but I was overwhelmed with gratitude for the insights that the visit had allowed.

I saw what we had done. Paul and Shannon loved their son. He was healthy and happy. Their lives were better because of Logan. He was a gift that they obviously treasured. I understood that now.

I was also overwhelmed with a sense of comprehension. I got it now.

Your job was to give this gift. Now your role is to stand back and watch Logan grow from afar.

All of the grief, pain, and tears were worth it because of this child. And even though we may never be part of his life, he will always be part of ours. The pain of his loss may never leave us, but it will eventually be conquered by love.

Sean and I will walk on, searching for answers that we may never have. We will overturn stones and move mountains to channel our grief in a more productive direction, and the strength to do this will come from love—the love we have for one another, and the love we have for our children. All four of them.

I closed my eyes and whispered a prayer to Logan.

Your birth was a blessing. Your life is a gift. And your mama and daddy love you very, very much. I've seen it with my own eyes and felt it with my own heart, so I know it is true. Sleep tight, Little One. Godspeed.

EPILOGUE

A Letter to Logan

September 24, 2010

Dear Logan,

It's hard to imagine that this time last year I was in the operating room, waiting eagerly for you to take your first breath. The moment you were born was one of the most joyous of my life. I will never forget how happy I was when I heard your first cry, and how relieved I was when Sean held your sweet face to mine and the nurse told me that you were perfectly healthy. It was in that moment that I knew you would never leave my heart. And you haven't.

It amazes me how often I think of you. In the first moments of my day, when I'm reviewing my "to-do" list, you creep in to my thoughts. I say a prayer for you then, hoping that the day brings you peace, happiness and health; that your minutes are full of fun, love and adventure; and that maybe—just maybe— today will be a day that we get a message about your progress.

As I tackle the routine of my day, you are with me. Sometimes when I'm packing lunches for our boys, I wonder what you like to eat. When I'm playing with MK, I wonder who is playing with you. I imagine how happy MK would have been to have you for a little brother. You two would have had great fun together. Those moments are sad for me, but I'm getting better at turning away from them. I don't have it mastered yet, but I hope someday the "what ifs" won't haunt me as often.

Amazingly, you've helped me through some tough times this past year. In January when the transfer of our two remaining embryos was unsuccessful and our chance to expand our family with our remaining embryos was lost, I relied on the thought of you to remind myself that some good came out of this. I know your parents and family love you very much and that they are happy that you are with them. We take solace in that.

Sean and I had a decision to make after our failed transfer. Do we try again? It was around then that we saw you for the second time, on national television. When we watched you that morning, sitting in your daddy's lap as your mommy gushed about how much you were loved, our yearning for another child overwhelmed us. Seeing you, inspired us. I have no idea whether our new doctor, and subsequent treatments will result in a child for our family, but we are grateful that you gave us the strength to move forward.

We still struggle. Sometimes, in the middle of the night, I see Sean sitting on the side of the bed staring out the window. I never ask what he is thinking. I already know. You see, night time is when we miss you the most. Sometimes, by staring up at the starry night, we comfort ourselves with the thought that that we are admiring the same sky that blankets you. Granted, the sky is vast, and you are far, far away, but it is one way that we feel connected to you. Right now, we'll take any connection with you we can have.

Sometimes I feel guilty for thinking of you so much. I know there are people who think it would be best if I could forget about you. Maybe it would be, but I can't. I have always understood the reason you are not being raised in our family. The hard part is that that logic has never translated to my heart.

I know now I wasn't cut out to be a gestational carrier. I just couldn't disconnect the way I needed to. I guess that is why it is so important that women who do become surrogates carefully consider their decision. I understand now what a difficult thing this is to do.

Most nights Sean and I go to sleep knowing nothing about how you're doing. Even though that is hard, we have kept our word. From the beginning, we told your parents that we would never intrude in their lives, or in yours. We thought that was the most generous way to move forward. We still stand by our promise to stay away unless invited, but want you to know that our absence says nothing about our love for you. Please never doubt that we care about you more than you could ever imagine.

Sometimes we think you are luckiest little boy in the whole world. You have two parents who treasure you, two sisters who adore you, and an extended family that, we imagine, are grateful for the gift of your life. And you have us too. Our door will always be open to you. If you ever need anything, as long as it doesn't interfere with your family, please know that we are here with open arms and loving hearts.

I hope you had a wonderful first birthday. I hope someone baked you a cake that you dug your chubby little fingers into, and that you made a glorious mess. I hope when they sang to you, you smiled brightly when you realized they were singing for you. I hope you opened a few gifts, but enjoyed the wrapping and the boxes more than the contents. And, most importantly, I hope you felt loved.

Happy birthday; sweet dreams; and Godspeed, Little Man. We will love your forever!

Carolyn and Sean

AFTERWORD

Carolyn and I struggled over how to proceed legally with the clinic that made this error. We had never been involved in a lawsuit before and wanted to keep it that way. But this clinic and its personnel hurt us in many ways. We also felt we had a duty to protect other patients of this or other clinics from a similar fate. If we avoided a suit and agreed not to disclose the name of the clinic or how the mistake happened, we would not be comfortable that we did everything to make sure this mistake would not be repeated at this facility or any other facility.

The legal process we pursued was a facilitation in which both parties engage each other through a third party to try to reach an agreement that prevents a lawsuit from being filed. We entered this process open-minded, but understood resolution might not come through facilitation. At our first facilitation in October, just weeks after delivery of Logan, we walked into the law firm of the facilitator and past the conference room where our fertility doctor sat. As we passed by the large windows of that conference room, Carolyn grabbed my hand and squeezed it tightly. I knew she would rather be anywhere else than in that place at that time. By the time we arrived at our conference room, she seemed ready to escape through the back door. The last time Carolyn and the doctor were this close he was performing the embryo transfer.

We spent five hours in the first facilitation, followed by two additional longer sessions in 2010. I think part of the strategy of these terribly long days is to motivate you to reach an agreement so that you can avoid ever having to go back. Each session produced a broad range of emotions from anger to sadness and, due to the absurdity of some of the legal arguments, even some humor. Following the third session some breakthroughs occurred and an agreement in principle was reached in May 2010. However, the process was far from over as it took well into November 2010 for the agreement to be signed by all parties.

As part of the settlement we agreed not to identify the clinic and the clinic agreed to pay us financial damages. The clinic also agreed to provide a full description of the mistake and how it was discovered as well as provide us documentation that it has implemented a revised protocol in its lab that would ensure that this mistake was never repeated. Written into the agreement was a clause that allowed Carolyn and I to release a summary of the medical mistake and revised protocol information to the public. We felt an obligation to share this with the IVF community including clinics, industry associations, current patients, and future patients.

Through this process Carolyn and I had to maintain a balance between protecting the public and having a level of compassion for the employees of the clinic. The professionals involved had spent their careers building an excellent reputation and we believed that they should continue to help couples have children.

The settlement did not feel like a victory to us. If anything, the process and ultimate resolution was sad and stressful and I am sure it was even more so for the clinic and our doctor. A settlement in a situation like this never gets you back to where you were before the mistake. We incurred massive costs that went well beyond expenses, stress that frequently took us to our knees, and lost time we will never get back with those around us, especially our children.

Carolyn and I will be tithing funds from the settlement and the proceeds from the book into a community foundation under the name of the Carolyn and Sean Savage Family. With our guidance, each year Drew and Ryan (and eventually Mary Kate) will help select worthy charitable causes for the foundation to support. When the appropriate day arrives, Logan will be invited to help us direct funds from the foundation.

HOW THE MISTAKE HAPPENED

FOR NEARLY EIGHTEEN MONTHS, Carolyn and I lived knowing another couple's embryos were transferred to Carolyn on February 6, 2009, but not knowing how the mistake was made or how it was discovered. Who was responsible? What went wrong? How did it get discovered? As part of a legal settlement in May 2010, the clinic's lawyers provided an explanation. A synopsis of that explanation follows:

- Upon initiating our frozen embryo transfer, an employee of the clinic completed a thaw order document that listed the name of our fertility doctor, our names, Carolyn's social security number, Carolyn's date of birth, my date of birth, and our phone number. Once the physician's staff forwarded the thaw order to the lab where the embryos were stored, the lab confirmed that it had received the order.
- With the order, an employee in the lab then printed labels containing all of the identifying information found on the thaw order. Every document pertaining to our frozen embryo transfer carried a label. *Important: These labels identified Carolyn's year of birth incorrectly.*
- The lab technician placed these labels on four pages called the patient jacket, an 11x17 sheet of paper folded in half. This jacket holds all the documents and laboratory notes on

the development of the embryos along with the thaw order
sheet, the receipt confirmation sheet and any leftover patient
identification labels.

- On February 2, 2009, five days before our transfer, the
embryologist used our identifying information on the thaw
order in our patient jacket to pull our Embryo Information
Sheet, a document that indicates the precise location of the
cryopreservation tank, the canister and the straws that house
our embryos. The clinic keeps their Embryo Information
Sheets on every patient in a large binder in the lab organized
alphabetically under the mother's name.

- This embryologist looked at the thaw order document in
our patient jacket, flipped to the "S" section of his binder,
and incorrectly pulled Shannon Savage's Embryo Information Sheet instead of Carolyn Savage's (Shannon used her
maiden name at the time of their original IVF procedure).
Using location information from Shannon Savage's Embryo
Information Sheet, he pulled Shannon Savage-Morell/
Paul Morell's embryos from the cryopreservation tank. Our
embryos remained in cryopreservation. The Embryo Information Sheet, the only paperwork that documents that the
embryos the embryologist pulled did not belong to Carolyn
and me, was placed in the back of the patient jacket.

- From that moment on, Shannon and Paul's embryos were
associated with Carolyn and my paperwork. Since the lab
associated their embryos with our paperwork, the name
Savage was written on the Petri dish and the canister stor-
ing the embryos. Our patient jacket was stored right next to
the canister holding the embryos. If anyone had checked the
Embryo Information Sheet in our patient jacket, they would
have found Shannon and Paul's Embryo Information Sheet.

- For the five days that the embryos thawed and grew in the
lab, the embryologist checked the embryos/labels against the

identifying information in the patient jacket. However, the embryos/labels were not checked against the Embryo Information Sheet inside the patient jacket.

- On the transfer day February 6, 2009, the embryologist walked into the procedure room where Carolyn was lying awaiting the transfer. He confirmed Carolyn's identity against the patient jacket he held in his hands.
- The doctor verbally confirmed that three embryos would be transferred. Then the embryologist delivered three of Paul and Shannon's embryos labeled with our names to the doctor. He also delivered the patient jacket to our doctor at this time.
- The doctor, trusting these were our embryos, did not cross check the Embryo Information Sheet held in the patient jacket and immediately transferred three of Paul and Shannon's embryos to Carolyn.

An error by the embryologist of the lab initiated the wrong embryos being pulled and then an insufficient protocol failed to catch the original error in the subsequent five days the embryos grew in the lab before transfer. The initial error by the embryologist in pulling the wrong Embryo Information Sheet was the key misstep, but the fact is this piece of paper was inside a thin file next to the embryos in every step of the five day process, including the procedure room where the embryo transfer took place. In our opinion, those responsible for the mistaken transfer include everyone involved in the process from the moment the wrong Embryo Information Sheet was pulled February 2nd through the transfer February 6th. Any member of the clinic involved with establishing and monitoring the safety protocols for the clinic is also responsible. The clinic's protocol was not sufficient and this is evidenced by the fact that the clinic changed its safety protocol on February 16, 2009, the day after the error was discovered.

The change was made too late for us, but fortunately not too late for future patients. Under the clinic's new protocol, in the event that two patients have the same last name, the staff affixes a bright orange sticker to the data sheets in the binder to alert personnel. The clinic created a "Patient Verification Form" that has multiple confirmations of patient identification information. Labels on the canes and straws containing the embryos now have five identifiers. The new protocol requires that the staff check all five identifiers before proceeding to the next step. The physician him/herself double checks all identifying information before completing the transfer. Initial documents are cross-checked, not just recently produced documents.

When our clinic discovered this weakness in their protocol, they conducted a review of patient records to be certain that they had made no other mistakes. By doing this, they confirmed that this was the only time that they had transferred the wrong embryos. Thankfully no one else they treated received our fate.

HOW WAS THE MISTAKE DISCOVERED?

OUR SETTLEMENT AGREEMENT ALSO required that the clinic describe how the error was discovered. Upon reading the description of the discovery my stomach sank and I had to read it again to make sure I was not mistaken. The explanation is outlined below.

- On Sunday, February 15, 2009, a clinic employee was doing data entry work into a computer regarding all transfers from the previous two weeks when a discrepancy in Carolyn's year of birth was discovered. Her label wrongly indicated that Carolyn was born in 1967 when her correct year of birth is 1969 and this caused the employee some confusion. To confirm the correct date of birth he decided to dig deeper and he paged through the patient jacket and found Shannon Savage's Embryo Information Sheet in the back of Carolyn's patient jacket.

- The employee immediately called the embryologist who came to the lab and soon discovered the error. The embryologist contacted Shannon's physician who in turn called our doctor.
- Our doctor then waited until Carolyn's positive pregnancy test the next day to inform us of the error.

The birth year being incorrect on the labels and Carolyn's wristband had *nothing* to do with Paul and Shannon's embryos being transferred to Carolyn. The birth year being incorrect was an independent error. Thus, it took a second mistake to discover the first mistake. Had Carolyn's year of birth been noted correctly, the wrong embryos would still have been transferred, but the error would not have been discovered on February 15th. The error probably would have gone undetected until Paul and Shannon would have decided to go through with a frozen embryo transfer. At that time the embryologist would have gone to pull their Embryo Information Sheet from the binder and it would have been missing. Likely, he'd then go to the cryopreservation tank and would have discovered that Paul and Shannon's embryos were missing. We do not know when this discovery would have been made.

I have been told the likelihood of the wrong embryos being transferred is one in three million. What are the chances that an independent error would have been made in conjunction with the same patient that would lead back to the original mistake? This is truly inconceivable.

Carolyn and I struggled with how or if to forgive while we dealt with the impact of the clinic's actions. Kevin Anderson helped us by introducing the idea of intolerant forgiveness: the ability to forgive the person who committed the error, but not the actual mistake. But while Carolyn was still pregnant, we couldn't embrace the idea as there was so much else on our minds. After Logan's birth and our movement into the next phase of acceptance of what had just happened to us, we focused more attention on how we would deal with the clinic on multiple fronts, including how or if we could ever forgive.

As the legal facilitation process played out, we learned through the mediator that our doctor was visibly distraught. His attorney communicated his deep sorrow for everything surrounding the mistake and the impact it had on our lives. His ongoing struggle with guilt and regret and the sincerity with which he communicated those feelings moved us. Yet our feelings about him were deeply conflicted. All along we knew his expertise and skill brought us Mary Kate when, for more than a decade, everyone else in his field had failed. We felt compassion for his suffering and thankfulness for his expertise with Mary Kate, but we also felt continued anger at him for introducing such a cross to bear in our lives.

We believe in having compassion for those who hurt us. Frequently, we fall short, but we needed to help him and all of those in the clinic to move on from this incident. Just as we had written a letter to him on February 18th, we felt compelled to do the same in January 2011.

Dear Doctor,

On numerous occasions we received your messages of deep sorrow and remorse that we understand is shared by several individuals in the clinic. We know these messages are heartfelt and they motivated us to send you this note.

We forgive you and everyone involved in the clinic who is seeking forgiveness. We cannot excuse the act, but we do have compassion for everyone who has to live with this mistake every day. Please release yourself of any guilt and move on with your life. You have much good to do with your career and your family.

Sincerely,
Carolyn and Sean Savage

ACKNOWLEDGMENTS

This book would not have been possible without the amazing work of our collaborating writer, Danelle Morton. Danelle, thank you for your countless hours of shaping, editing, and writing! Your insights and keen eye for how to arrange a well-told story have been priceless, and your patience and grace through the challenging moments did not go unnoticed. We are especially grateful for the way you motivated us to write through the most painful of memories. You said we'd be better for it. You were right. We cannot wait to see what you do next, as it seems that everything you touch turns to gold!

We owe a lifetime of gratitude to our literary agent, Linda Loewenthal of the David Black Agency. At a time when we were getting many calls, we had the good fortune of being referred to David, who listened, understood, and knew you'd be the best match for us. We are well aware that you went above and beyond for us throughout the entire process and were always our number one advocate. We have respect for your professionalism and expertise and admire your personal ethic. You are a blessing in our lives.

We knew from the minute we met with our editor Cindy DiTiberio and our entire team at HarperOne that we made an ideal match! Your insights into what we wanted to accomplish in this book were spot on and your valuable feedback made our story more poignant. Thank you for everything you did in helping us deliver our story to the world.

Thank you to Stephanie Siegel, Esther Zucker and Jackie Levin of NBC. You saw us as people first and a story second. Your professional approach helped us maintain our dignity while sharing our very personal story with the public. You are at the top of your profession.

We would not have been able to endure the challenges of this situation if it had not been for the love and support of our parents. It is the lessons we learned from you as children that shaped our choices of today. We both have talked about the moment when we realized you were not just our parents, but people. And, thankfully for us, you are the best kind of people. We can only hope that when our children are adults they have as much respect and love for us as we do you.

Family is where it all begins and our immediate and extended family is awesome. We are so fortunate to have so many relatives that care about us and support us through actions and prayer. We thank brothers, sisters, brother-in-laws, sister-in-laws, aunts, uncles, cousins and all of those family members who have gone before us. Your support carried us and your prayers lifted us. We will never forget.

This journey deeply challenged us on an emotional level. We would not be "getting through" without the assistance of our therapist, Dr. Kevin Anderson. Kevin, your kind-hearted spirit and ability to reign in our emotions to a place of meaning and respect, have only improved our lives. The lessons of love, compassion, and empathy have enriched us in a way that we could have never imagined.

We will be eternally grateful for the compassionate and topnotch care we received from Dr. Elizabeth Reid and her staff at Premier Women's Health. We want you all to know that whenever we entered your office, we knew that you cherished Logan's life as much as we did. We are positive that he would not be in this world today without your expertise.

We are also grateful to the entire medical team and staff at Mercy St. Vincent Medical Center. You made sure that Logan entered this world safely, and honored our role in his life with humanity. His birth gave us the only moment we will ever have as his mom and dad, and your arrangements provided us with priceless memories. As healers, your care and love brought us dignity and comfort when we needed it most.

In our desperate search for a new fertility clinic and home for our embryos, we were lucky to find Dr. Robert Straub and the entire staff of Reproductive Biology Associates of Atlanta, Georgia. Thank you for taking such good care of us and Jennifer during our time in treatment.

We would also like to thank the faculty and staff of St. Johns Jesuit High School and St. Joseph School, Sylvania, for ministering to our boys throughout this journey. We are so appreciative of the way you kept the boys on track academically and anticipated their emotional needs during a very challenging time. We are truly blessed to have you as partners in educating our children.

Father Joseph Cardone was our first call after learning of our pregnancy with Logan. Fr. Cardone, you helped us calm our fears on a day that we found ourselves in a state of unimaginable shock. We truly appreciate the wisdom you imparted on us and we are also grateful for your ministry throughout our journey. We are lucky to call you a friend.

We had four gifted and caring attorneys that helped us navigate our way through a tangled web of communication, legal precedent, and critical decision making. Mary Smith, your care and concern with our emotional as well as legal well-being was very much appreciated. We couldn't have prepared for what this pregnancy would bring us without the cool head and valuable insights of

Marty Holmes Sr. Of course, our third call the evening of February 16, 2009, was to our trusted friend, Marty Holmes Jr. Marty you walked this journey with us long past Logan's delivery as not only a valued attorney but more importantly, a friend. Thank you so much for your compassionate and smart advice, loyalty and support. Lastly, we were blessed to be under the competent care of Brian McKeen of McKeen and Associates. Brian, you cared about us first and the legal case second. You are at the top of your profession, and yet enthusiastically accessible at all times. We admire your strong convictions and the honorable way you advocate for your clients.

One of the greatest supports during the pregnancy came from a very special group of women . . . The Reliable Girls (Beth, Julie, Kim, Laurel, Lynn, Melissa, Nancy, Suzanne and Tracy). The fact that we met an unconventional manner is what had made our friendship and your support so special. You were always there, sometimes many times a day. We will be eternally grateful for your thoughtful counsel, and heartfelt compassion. Whatever you need, whenever you need it, just say the word!

Our friends are the best! We couldn't have faced this challenge without them. We'd like to especially thank Ann Mancinotti, Tracy Kindl, Kathleen Nowak, Linda Steinberg, Rachel Kalas, Mary Jo Jacoby, Craig Bruning, Matt Dzierwa, Greg Periatt, Tony Desch, Dan Hartnett, Steve and Ellen Baugh, Mike and Anne White and the many other friends who helped and supported us. We love all of you.

There is not a doubt in our minds that Logan is loved by Paul and Shannon Morell. Paul and Shannon, we are incredibly grateful for the two visits we have had with Logan since his birth. The occasional updates and pictures that you send also bring us some much needed peace of mind. We know that this journey has been difficult for you. Even though we have no idea what the future holds for any of us, please know that you will always be welcome in our home. We wish only the best for your family.

The lights of our lives are Drew, Ryan, and Mary Kate. Kids, we love you more than words can say and we are grateful for the blessings you have brought into our lives. When times are tough, you have no idea how your successes, smiles, giggles, or calm conversations bring us peace and happiness. Your futures hold so much promise. We thank God every day for the gift of your lives.

Inconceivable Choices

There are times in everyone's lives when they have to make difficult choices. Whether by a fateful accident, or circumstances self-created or brought about by another, somehow you are faced with a choice that you will need to live with for the rest of your life. These types of choices can be wide ranging: from fertility problems, aging parents, medical crises, career crises, marital issues, to parenting challenges. These are moments when the world seems askew. When facing these inconceivable choices, you need as much help and support as you can find. Support can come from your faith, or from those you know and trust, but it can also come from those you have yet to meet.

For us, the defining moment on this journey came on February 16, 2009 when we learned about this inconceivable medical mistake and made the choice not to terminate the pregnancy , nor to fight for custody of Logan after he was born. In the aftermath of those choices, we leaned on our faith, counselors, family, and friends for support. Help also came in a nontraditional manner: Carolyn found a group of women online who had faced infertility problems. Her "Reliable Girls" were spread around the United States and Canada but their support was as constant and immediate as if they were living around the corner. We also tapped into other online resources to answer our many questions. Our experiences inspired us to build an online community specifically designed to support people who are facing difficult choices. That community is growing right now at inconceivablechoices.com.

We welcome you to this community if you are facing a difficult choice or if you want to provide input and support to other members. We have also invited experts in specific disciplines including counselors, psychologists, psychiatrists, spiritual leaders, and professors to provide advice on issues the community is facing. The various points of view both from these experts as well as other members will benefit members of the community while they are deciding their course of action, as well as support and compassion in the aftermath of their choices.

Our vision for this community is that it will inspire regular people like us to do the right thing, which in turn will benefit our world. We will be at inconceivablechoices.com trying to help and seeking support as well. Please join us.